A CURE FOR CROHN'S

The Untold Cause and Emerging Treatment for Crohn's Disease

Dr. David N. Armstrong

Published by: Armstrong Medical Inc., Atlanta GA. ArmstrongMed@gmail.com

ISBN: 978-1-7371333-1-5 (e)
ISBN: 978-1-7371333-0-8 (sc, B&W)
ISBN: 978-1-7371333-2-2 (hc, B&W)
ISBN:978-1-7371333-3-9 (sc, color)
ISBN:978-1-7371333-4-6 (hc, color)

Library of Congress Control Number: 2021910172

*This book is dedicated to all patients with Crohn's disease.
And to Toby, one of my young patients who took his own life owing
to this devastating disease.*

TABLE OF CONTENTS

INTRODUCTION

I am probably the only colorectal surgeon that has seen a cow die of Johne's (pronounced Yo-nee's) disease, a chronic intestinal wasting disease in cattle. Since there are only a couple of thousands of us in the US, that's not a stretch.

I *know* I am the only colorectal surgeon who has looped a winch cable around the dead cow's front hooves, signaled to the winch operator to haul her into the knacker wagon, see her neck break as she is hauled through the narrow byre door, and hear the sickening crack when her hind leg is trapped under the ramp as the merciless winch drags her into a pile of dead sheep, pigs, and cows. A cargo of death. The stench is unbelievable. It's supposed to be: An ethereal warning from the dead to the living: "Stay away from us. Something is terribly wrong." I could never understand why the knacker man did this for a living or why he always seemed to be so happy doing his job. People ask me the same question.

The "knacker man" trade has been around for centuries, for as long as animals have been kept on farms. He is the critical guardian who keeps dead animals that are unfit for human consumption away from living livestock to be sold at auction, on the way to the dinner plate. The knacker man's dead animals are rendered into soap, glue, fertilizer, bone meal, animal food, hides. Nothing is left to waste. Nothing. It's not pretty. It never was. It never will be.

Just like humans, every cow has a personality. There are angry cows, who will try to kick you in the face as you bend down to place the suction cups onto her teats at "milking time." Cows kick forward with their hind legs to protect their udders. Horses kick back. You can stand behind the hind legs of the craziest cow, and you are safe. If you stand behind the hind legs of a crazy horse, you may end up dead. There are docile cows, who swish their tails and chew their fodder as you put cups on their teats. There are greedy cows, who head butt their sisters away from the fodder or water trough as they eat and drink their fill. There are shy cows who graze by themselves, away from the herd. There are even "horny" cows, who mount their sisters when they are in heat—so-called "bulling." This is a sure sign to call for Artificial Insemination (AI), to have her inseminated by bull semen of the farmer's choice to propagate the herd. The life of a 21st-century cow is not particularly exciting.

When the dead cow is winched from the byre, all the cows turn quiet. There is no fighting, no head-butting, no kicking, and no "humping." Nobody competes for the fodder or the water trough. Like silent mourners at a funeral, they turn away in silence. The message always gets through.

In the past, I always wanted to be a veterinary surgeon. The local vet was none other than the legendary author James Herriot, in Thirsk, 25 miles away from the farm. Author of *All Creatures Great and Small, All Things Bright and Beautiful,* and *If Only They Could Talk,* he was a local hero. The TV series and movies based on his books were filmed in the local Yorkshire Dales. Beautiful, undulating in summer; harsh and unforgiving in winter. Anyway, instead, I went to medical school and became a surgeon, to learn to operate on that most fractious and unpredictable animal—man.

I had no idea, decades later, as a colorectal surgeon, that I would see Johne's disease again, this time masquerading under a different name—Crohn's disease.

Had I not seen Johne's disease first hand on the farm, I still may have read, somewhere, that Johne's disease is caused by a bacterium, Mycobacterium Avium Paratuberculosis (MAP), which is carried by swarms of migrating birds, contaminating the pasturelands below and causing Johne's disease in cattle. I may or may not have understood that Johne's- infected cattle secrete MAP in their milk[1] and contaminate consumer milk supplies, including baby formula[2]. MAP-contaminated milk then causes Johne's disease in humans. But now the name changes to Crohn's disease.

I may have read, somewhere, that MAP is transmitted in cow's milk to their suckling calves, causing Johne's disease. I probably would not have realized that MAP is also transmitted in the breast milk[3] of Crohn's disease patients to their nursing infants, thereby causing Crohn's disease. If I had never seen Johne's disease on the farm, I may not have been particularly interested in, or even understood, the connection between Johne's disease and Crohn's disease. If we need to thank anyone or anything for stirring my interest, we need look no further than my Crohn's patients - and, of course, the cow.

Crohn's disease is Johne's disease and Johne's disease is Crohn's disease. They are one and the same. There is no daylight between them[4].

For decades, the medical community has labeled Crohn's disease as "idiopathic." Aka, "we don't know." Like every other "idiopathic" disease, Crohn's disease is treated with steroids, which help in the short term, but cannot be used indefinitely. Treating diseases we don't know the cause of with medications we don't know the mechanism of is an old favorite in medicine. It's called "empiric" therapy. (It is a disappointingly short name for a medical term, but stay tuned.) Nevertheless, somehow, it usually works out. Biologics (Humira, Remicade, Cimzia, Stelera, Entyvio) target "immune modulators," the "interleukins," and dampen the immune response. They definitely help, often dramatically. But like steroids, they treat the results of the disease, the massive inflammatory response, but not the underlying cause of Crohn's. Biologics are massively expensive, often tens of thousands of dollars per dose, and when the medication is stopped, usually because patients lose their health insurance, Crohn's disease returns. With a vengeance.

Veterinarians have known for a hundred years that Johne's disease is caused by MAP[5], but only in the last few years has evidence emerged that MAP also causes Crohn's disease. Even now, the debate is contentious, bordering on schizophrenic. It is not taught in medical school, residency, or fellowship programs. When I explain the link to colleagues or my colorectal fellows I get "the look"—"nut job."

The Johne's-Crohn's connection is a real-life medical mystery[6]. There are numerous unexplained Crohn's "coincidences" throughout the world, "hotspots" and "clusters" which defy conventional medical logic. Why did twelve children in a single street in Winnipeg develop Crohn's disease out of the blue?[7] Why is Crohn's disease in Australian children escalating, when the disease was previously unknown?[8] Why, in the 1990s, did the rate of Crohn's disease in Iceland increase by a factor of twenty, from a standing start?[9] Why did Crohn's disease become a mini epidemic in Czechoslovakia, thirty years after independence from the USSR?[10] Why did twelve children in a French village all develop Crohn's disease, within a few years of each other?[11] Why did seven unrelated pupils at the Mankato[12], MN Class of 1980 simultaneously develop Crohn's disease?

A Cure for Crohn's addresses an extremely complex and controversial topic. It is divided into four parts, as much for my understanding and comprehension as it is for the reader, new to the topic. Part one outlines the whole Johne's-Crohn's controversy and my own immersion into the enigma, including the cow. Part two tracks MAP's great-grandfather, tuberculosis (Mycobacterium tuberculosis), which was integrally tied to Johne's and Crohn's disease and was inextricably entwined into the enigma. MAP's surname is, after all, "paratuberculosis," a proud member of a historic lineage of serial killers[6]. The scramble for an antibiotic against tuberculosis occasionally resulted in an unforeseen spin-off, an afterthought, which resulted in an antibiotic that was effective against MAP. The only reason we have antibiotics that are effective against MAP and Crohn's disease is because of the war against tuberculosis.

Smallpox, the sister pandemic to tuberculosis, is tied into the story with Zabdiel Boylston's (after the Boston Street) first mass immunization campaign in man. Smallpox's ancient cousin, cowpox, is integrally tied into this convoluted, twisted fable. We trace Louis Pasteur's battle to sterilize milk (pasteurization) against tuberculosis, but it ultimately falls short in killing MAP and preventing transmission of Johne's and Crohn's diseases.

Part three starts to shed light on MAP, Johne's and Crohn's diseases and, by a series of lucky breaks, we start to unravel the threads of the mystery. Part four tracks the chaotic and cut-throat campaigns for new antibiotics to treat mankind's killers—tuberculosis, streptococcus, staphylococcus, E Coli, and, eventually, MAP and Crohn's disease. In the last few years, a paradigm shift has emerged. Crohn's disease, like Johne's disease, is caused by a bacterium (MAP) and can be treated successfully and effectively with antibiotics. This may not seem a stretch; it just took a hundred years for us to reach that conclusion. The first "Crohn's antibiotic" is being developed by Tel Aviv's RedHill Biopharma, an antibiotic cocktail designated RHB-104. It is by complete coincidence that a few months ago, in December 2020, the final results of the first phase 3 study of RHB-104 in treating Crohn's disease were reported on the website: www.clinicaltrails.gov. The study results were a blockbuster success. RHB-104 is the first designated Crohn's antibiotic. It has broken the mold that Crohn's disease is an "idiopathic" disease of cause unknown; that treatment for Crohn's must be "empiric"— a "blunderbuss" approach. Finally, we have a targeted antibiotic treatment for a known bacterium that causes a known disease. We should not be shocked that it actually works. RHB-104 may have broken the mold as the first antibiotic regimen for Crohn's disease, but it will not be the last.

I have many people to thank for this book. Fred Quinn, Professor of Infectious Diseases at University of Georgia College of Veterinary Medicine in Athens, GA, a few miles away from my surgical practice, provided crucial insight into Johne's disease. Unsolicited, he offered the resources of his lab to delve into the topic deeper and at no cost.

Dr. Rodrick Chiodini, prolific MAP researcher and outspoken campaigner of the Johne's-Crohn's connection, was generous with his time and experience in his long quest. He also offered valuable insight, such as a pivotal meeting between the United States Department of Agriculture (USDA) and MAP researchers (himself included), when all cellphones were collected at the door, and a list of permitted questions was handed to meeting participants.

Finally, and by no means least, is the owner/operator of one of the largest and most up-to-date robotic daily farms in the UK. This individual happens to be my cousin, Robert Armstrong, in Arrathorne, North Yorkshire, who established one of the largest, most sophisticated robotic dairy farms in Europe. Fully automated and incredibly efficient, the robot dairy farm automatically milks hundreds of cows, 24 hours a day. Enticed by an endless supply of fodder, the cows compete to enter the stalls. Their udders are sterilized by a laser-guided spray, the cups are applied by a robotic arm, and milk output is carefully monitored—wirelessly—until all four udders are adequately milked. Monitored by computer, the process is safe, efficient, and the cutting edge of dairy farming. If any cow shows signs of dwindling milk production—the earliest sign of possible Johne's disease, the cow is isolated and screened. The bulk milk is analyzed daily for MAP to prevent the MAP-Johne's-Crohn's chain. The operation is the future of the dairy industry and a key step in the prevention of Crohn's disease.

This book relays the story of Crohn's disease. It relates the long and complex journey to where we are now. The heroes of the saga, the villains, the breakthroughs, the flashes of genius, the tragedies, and the occasional lucky breaks. Finally, the evidence is presented to you, the jury, to render a verdict in the hope that understanding the link between MAP and this terrible disease may spur interest, acceptance, understanding, and, most importantly, much more research. In the words of Thomas Jefferson, "Knowledge is power."

PART ONE: ZOONOSIS DENIED

*Oxford English dictionary: 1631/1 Zoonosis, (noun).
Any disease communicated or communicable from one of
the lower animals to man. Late 19th century from zoo -'of
animals' + Greek nosos 'disease'.*

CHAPTER 1

FROM BIRDS TO COWS TO MAN

Crohn's disease (CD) is a chronic, debilitating intestinal disease that affects an estimated five million people worldwide, including over 1.5 million Americans. Its incidence is increasing rapidly, and it disproportionately affects children, adolescents, and young adults. An inflammatory disease, Crohn's causes inflammation anywhere throughout the intestinal tract: in the small bowel, where nutrients are absorbed; the large bowel (colon), where water and electrolytes are absorbed; and even the rectum and perianal area. In the small bowel, Crohn's may cause strictures, which is when the small intestine narrows. This narrowing can result in excruciating abdominal pain, bowel obstruction, uncontrollable vomiting, and dramatic weight loss. In addition to strictures, Crohn's can lead to holes, or perforations, in the tissue wall, which are life-threatening and require immediate surgery. As a life-saving measure, surgery frequently involves bringing a loop of bowel to the skin surface (a "stoma") to control spillage of stool into the abdominal cavity. Many of these stomas are required lifelong and are a constant source of diminished self-image and a burden to an active life in otherwise healthy adolescents.

In the colon, Crohn's disease can lead to intractable diarrhea, bleeding, abdominal cramps, and again, possibly perforation, and likely a colostomy, often lifelong. Inflammation anywhere in the bowel can result in one part of the intestine rupturing to an adjacent loop, causing an abnormal connection or fistula. This causes worsening pain, more dramatic weight loss, and uncontrolled diarrhea. Patients with uncontrolled Crohn's are typically bone-thin, wasted, pale, and emaciated.

Lastly, Crohn's disease can affect the tissues around the rectum, causing massive inflammation, abscesses, and rupturing from the rectum to the outside skin—anal fistula. These fistulas are particularly aggressive, cause intolerable pain, and excruciating discomfort.

The cause of Crohn's disease—officially—is unknown.

There is no cure for Crohn's disease.

The available treatments are inadequate. At best.

The first line of treatment consists of steroids, the panacea of the 21st century. This simply dampens the inflammation and does little or nothing to reverse the course of the disease.

In addition to steroids, new biologics such as Humira and Remicade also reduce inflammatory changes and often achieve dramatic improvement. Unfortunately, the fix is temporary. Once the patient stops taking the medication, the disease returns.

Surgery for Crohn's disease is particularly difficult and dangerous. Due to the massive inflammation, abdominal surgery is risky and dangerous. Postoperative deaths are not infrequent. This is because the thickened bowel often results in the removal of large segments of intestinal tissue, which frequently worsens the diarrhea and weight loss. Additionally, inflammation leads to other complications. Massive inflammation makes the blood vessels particularly difficult to control, and many times in my 30-year career, I have been faced with torrential blood loss due to damage of a mesenteric (intestinal) vessel, resulting in near exsanguination hemorrhage.

In many ways, Crohn's disease is worse than colon cancer. Surgical resection of colon cancer is relatively simple and straightforward compared to surgery for Crohn's disease. Colon cancers are isolated, do not spread throughout the bowel, and, typically, are easily resected surgically.

But this is not the case in Crohn's disease.

Once the colon cancer has been resected, it rarely returns. But in the case of Crohn's disease, the question is often not *if* the disease will recur, but *when* and *where*. Many young Americans are faced with stomas (ileostomies or colostomies), wherein the bowel is brought to the surface of the skin as a last-ditch measure to save the patient's life.

Death from Crohn's disease is not uncommon. Death following Crohn's disease surgery is not rare. Unfortunately, there is very little federal funding in research for Crohn's disease. Primarily, research dollars are generated by the Crohn's and Colitis Foundation of America, a private charitable organization of relatives of patients with Crohn's, philanthropic individuals, and corporate donors.

There is a little known, but critically important, fact about Crohn's disease, a "backstory" to the whole tragedy. Crohn's disease also occurs in cattle, where it is known as "Johne's disease," (JD) after the German veterinarian Heinrich Albert Johne, who described the disease in 1895, Johne's disease is almost identical to Crohn's disease in whatever aspects of the diseases are examined[13]. The disease has been known for over a hundred years and has identical features in animals as it does in humans. Dairy cattle become wasted, milk production decreases, liquid diarrhea spills over the pasture, and the cow eventually dies a wasting death, if not culled first. Importantly, the intestinal findings in Johne's disease are identical to Crohn's disease. Just as there is in Crohn's, intestinal narrowing, fistulas, and inflammation are frequent in Johne's.

If someone were to compare bowel tissue affected with Crohn's and Johne's disease under a microscope, they would see a very similar picture. In fact, the diagnostic hallmark which clinches a diagnosis of Crohn's disease—a cluster of inflammatory cells known as a "granuloma" —is also found in Johne's disease. The inflamed lining of the bowel, the mucosa, has a "cobblestone" appearance, and is a constant feature of both diseases. The inflammation can rupture through the bowel to an adjacent organ to cause fistulas, a characteristic of both Crohn's and Johne's disease. If the gut ruptures into the abdominal cavity, peritonitis ensues, requiring immediate emergency surgery in humans, and, for cattle, a merciful culling or an excruciating death awaits.

The origin of Crohn's disease is officially "idiopathic," i.e., "unknown". However, it has been known for over a hundred years that Johne's disease, the human equivalent of Crohn's disease, is caused by a bacterium, *Mycobacterium avium paratuberculosis*, or MAP. In Johne's disease, swarms of MAP can be seen in the intestine. Using various stains and conditions, cultures of MAP are visible under a microscope. MAP is endemic to migrating birds that overfly the pasture lands of Scandinavia, northern Europe, and North America. Carried by flocks of migrating birds, principally the starling, MAP contaminates pasture grasses through bird droppings, which are then ingested by grazing dairy cattle. Fun fact: *avium* is Latin for "bird," hence the name *Mycobacterium avium paratuberculosis*. MAP enters the intestinal tract of the dairy cattle, where it inflicts intestinal inflammation, narrowing, strictures, and perfo-ration. Meanwhile, the cow dies a slow, wasting death, spraying her MAP-infected liquid stool around the pastures, to be ingested by the remaining herd. MAP is also secreted in the cow's milk[1], and enters the consumer milk supply in the form of raw liquid milk[14], pasteurized milk[15, 16], cream, yogurt, cheese, and other milk prod-ucts[17], including baby formula[2]. To make matters worse, Johne's disease is consistently passed on to the next generation.[13,16] After giving birth to a calf, a Johne's-infected cow transmits her MAP-infected milk to her suckling newborn, guaranteeing a new gen-eration of MAP-infected cattle. Furthermore, numbers are steadily rising in both North America and Europe, and strict testing, isola-tion, and culling programs have had little impact.

Likewise, it is now known that patients with Crohn's disease also have intestinal tissue riddled with MAP "spheroplasts"[18], cell-wall deficient MAP bacteria, invisible to conventional microscopy. These "invisible" spheroplasts were a critical point of contention in the Johne's-Crohn's furor for decades[18–20].

About a century ago, Crohn's was found mostly in Scandinavia, Northern Europe, and occasionally in North America. Not only is it increasing rapidly in these original locations, but in recent decades, it is also spreading to nations hitherto untouched, includ-ing Iceland[9], Australia[8], and New Zealand[21], where the disease primarily targets children[22–24]. These regions have reported dra-matic spikes in the disease. The story repeats itself time after time. Figure 1 illustrates the migration and density maps of the common starling (Starling vulgaris). Historically, the bird was indigenous to Scandinavia and northern Europe, until it was introduced, by man, into and North America, Australia, New Zealand, and South Africa to protect crops against insect infestation. The birds carried along with them their indigenous bacterium, MAP, which caused

Johne's disease in the local cattle herds and eventually Crohn's disease in the resident population. Figure 2. illustrates the results of this: The global map of Crohn's disease, the highest prevalence in Scandinavia, Northern Europe, North America, Australia, New Zealand, and South Africa. The incidence of Crohn's disease and the density of Starling vulgaris (Figure 3) and Johne's disease (Figure 4) are basically a "copy and paste", a "cause and effect" of the link between MAP and Crohn's disease.

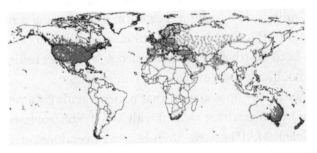

Figure 1. Global Starling prevalence map. Win Kirkpatrick, 2007.
Department of Primary Industries and Regional Development.
Government of Western Australia. Reproduced with permission.

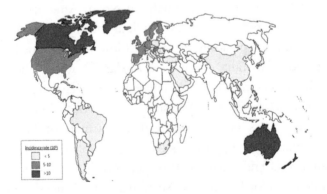

Figure 2. Global prevalence of Crohn's disease.
Ng S. et al. Gut 2013. Reproduced with permission.

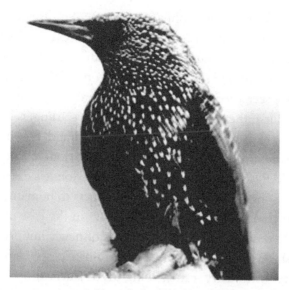

Figure 3. Starling vulgaris.

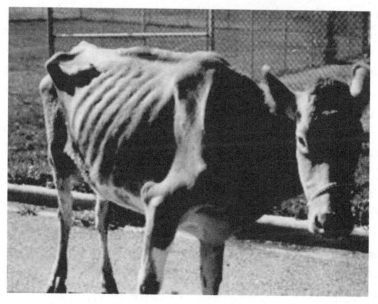

Figure 4. Johne's disease in cows.

Crohn's disease, like Johne's, is a zoonotic disease[4,5] That is, it transmits from birds to animals to humans. Transmission from birds to cows and eventually to humans can take several paths, and evidence from around the world suggests one of three possible scenarios. One scenario implicates an avian (bird) source as the initiating event: First, the carrier of the disease, the starling, is introduced to a region—for example, Australia, New Zealand, South Africa—as a measure against pest control. The avian source (the starling) spreads MAP over the grasslands and causes Johne's disease in cattle, which is then transmitted in milk products to humans, resulting in Crohn's disease. In a second scenario, as in the case of Iceland[9], the disease was introduced by thousands of newly imported MAP-infected sheep in the 1930s. Sheep contaminate pasturelands, which they share with dairy cattle, with MAP-laden droppings. The MAP-laden grass is consumed by dairy cattle, which causes Johne's disease, and is duly transmitted to humans, causing Crohn's disease. In a third scenario, as in the case of the newly independent Czechoslovakia, MAP came directly with imported Johne's-infected cattle from Western Europe. Johne's disease propagates to the indigenous, native cattle, and MAP spreads unseen in the cattle herds and milk supply. In each and all scenarios, the incidence of Johne's disease in cattle spikes and the cases of Crohn's disease skyrocket in the native population, mostly children.

Uncovering MAP in Human Crohn's Disease

Unfortunately, MAP is a very difficult bacterium to identify and isolate. The bacteria have a thick, waxy coat, which is difficult to stain using conventional stains, and is notoriously difficult to culture, requiring specific culture mediums at very specific temperatures. The MAP bacteria are "disappearing artists" and masters of disguise.

The initial studies into the link between MAP and Crohn's disease, therefore, failed to identify the bacteria in Crohn's disease tissues, and the theory was regarded as bogus and a scaremongering stunt. In conventional strains of Crohn's tissues, MAP was invisible, and anxious researchers, therefore, drew a blank. There was no "smoking gun." The glove didn't fit. For the detractors, this was the ultimate nail in the coffin of the "MAP alarmists" who were causing growing public alarm about the safety of milk products.

In 1989, a breakthrough occurred. Dr. Rodrick Chiodini (Figure 5) at Brown University, an outspoken veteran of the MAP theory, provided critical evidence by feeding biopsy samples from a young girl with Crohn's disease ("Linda") to newborn goats[25]. Eventually, after many months, the young goats receiving the "Linda" specimen developed the equivalent of Crohn's disease. Call it Johne's or Crohn's, it is the same disease in animals and man.

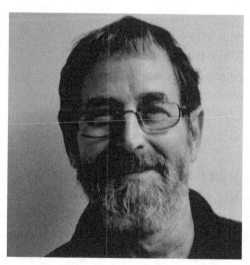

Figure 5. Professor Rodrick Chiodini.

MAP is often referred to as the master of disguise because it is invisible to stains. Fortunately, it has one dead giveaway: its DNA. The presence of a DNA sequence known as IS900 was eventually isolated using polymerase chain reaction (PCR). This DNA sequence is unique to MAP[26]. Armed with their new weapon, researchers reexamined Crohn's disease tissues, and IS900 sequences were present in nearly 100% of samples[27]. It was even found circulating in the bloodstream of subjects with Crohn's. Most alarmingly, it was found in the breast milk of mothers with Crohn's disease[28], who were unwittingly transferring the deadly bacterium to their newborn[29]. Several years later, Dr. Chiodini went on to provide the critical explanation for the invisible MAP. On entering the human body, the MAP bacterium sheds its thick, waxy coat and becomes an invisible ghost of a bacterium. Technically, it is called a spheroplast in the scientific community[18]. The parasitic spheroplast hides within the victim's own cells, where it steals nutrients and energy and hides away from the marauding immune system circulating outside.

This evidence was irrefutable. This was a cold case solved[3,4]. Crohn's and Johne's were the same disease[30]. Nonetheless, in a desperate attempt to protect the industry, the United States Department for Agriculture (USDA) and the powerful dairy lobby refused (and still refuse) to accept this and continued to regard the whole notion as a conspiracy theory and alarmist[31].

The Challenge of Research into MAP and Crohn's Disease

The initial MAP-Crohn's controversy, early failures to detect MAP in Crohn's tissues, and the public scare over milk safety—all have resulted in federal funding being virtually nonexistent. Most of the funding is from the Crohn's & Colitis Foundation (CCFA), people with Crohn's, their families' individual donations, and the occasional philanthropist. Because of the lack of federal funding, a few outspoken and largely ignored individuals have taken up the mantle to advocate for these patients and demand further funding and research. The notion that Crohn's disease is caused by MAP has been suppressed by government authorities across the world, primarily in the US and Europe. This is not taught in any medical school, and even veteran surgeons and gastroenterologists look puzzled and suspicious when I explain the link between Johne's and Crohn's disease[3,32]. Perhaps it is due to the initial evidence being controversial and possibly a result of social and political pressures. Government agencies continue to dismiss the theory. The European Union has published a 56-page, 376 reference position paper, stating there is "insufficient evidence to confirm or disprove" the link between MAP and Crohn's disease.[33]

Daphne E Thompson, a Government Biochemist and writing on behalf of the UK Department of Health,[20] concluded that the link could not be "proved or disproved." In the US, the major detractors are the USDA, who are carefully protecting the influential mega-dairy and milk industry. Additionally, the Centers for Disease Control and Prevention (CDC) denies any association. As a real-time confirmation of this, go to www.CDC.gov and enter "Crohn's disease and Mycobacterium Paratuberculosis" in the "search" engine. Nothing too controversial. Of the 155 results and 13 pages of results that populate this search, there is no mention whatsoever about MAP and Crohn's disease. Understandably suspicious, the medical establishment remains skeptical.

Because of low funding, a MAP vaccine is being developed single-handedly by Professor Herman Taylor (Figure 6) a retired surgeon in London, who has been a lone voice in the wilderness developing a vaccine for the treatment and prevention of MAP and Crohn's disease. Headquartered from his website (www.HAV-vaccine.com), funded by private investors and with collaboration from the Jenner Institute of Oxford University, progress on the vaccine remains slow. Unfortunately, the latest clinical trial for patients with Crohn's disease is on hold due to the Covid-19 epidemic.

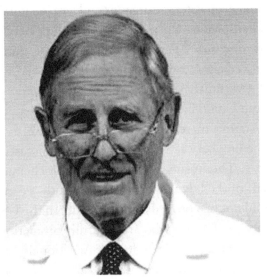

Figure 6. Professor John Hermon-Taylor.

Early antibiotic trials in treating MAP and Crohn's disease were unsuccessful since MAP was resistant to the standard anti-tuberculosis antibiotics studied. When antibiotics effective against MAP were tried, they met with stunning success. In Australia, Professor Thomas Borody, a gastroenterologist, developed a combination of three antibiotics, each effective against MAP. He found a dramatic reversal of Crohn's disease when subjects were treated with his antibiotic cocktail[34]. In combination with an Israeli company, RedHill Biopharma, the new drug, named RHB-104[35], has shown impressive treatment outcomes in individuals with Crohn's disease. This new data begs the question: if MAP is not the cause of Crohn's disease, why do antibiotics against MAP result in stunning successful outcomes, the likes of which any competing pharmaceutical company would give their right arm for?

With the United States Department of Agriculture (USDA) in opposition to the Johne's- Crohn's connection, with the Centers for Disease Control (CDC) in denial and with Food and Drug Administration (FDA) responsible for drug review, eventual approval of RHB-104 lies in doubt. The FDA, who ultimately would be responsible for approving registration for the medication in the US, may not wish to break step and may be unwilling to grant such authority. Meanwhile, 1.5 million American children and four million across the world, continue to suffer Crohn's disease without any curative medication[36]. Physicians, gastroenterologists, and surgeons like myself continue to patch up and piece together the broken remnants of children and young adults who are afflicted by this devastating disease and left in the wake of regulatory denial, administrative skepticism, and professional blindness.

CHAPTER 2

A DYING COW

A young boy stared at the wasted cow. He gazed in dismay at her bowed head, sagged in silent despair, her staring eyes sunk deep into their sockets, and her bare bones protruding through her ulcerated, matted hide. Because the fragile cow was too weak to stand, he and his father had made a makeshift rope harness, slung from the worm-infested roof timbers, in a desperate attempt to keep her upright. They both knew that once she lay down, she would surely die. The tiny, half-derelict cow byre leaked freezing rainwater that came down in torrents on the small farm huddled on the North Yorkshire moors. The solitary lightbulb, caked with years of bird droppings and matted with spider webs, cast a dark glow over the scene.

I turned to my father, looking strained and worried at the impending loss. One more dead cow. As pathetic and wretched as she was, she was part of a dwindling herd from which our family eked out a bare existence.

"What is it?" I asked.

Without turning, staring despairingly at the dying cow, he murmured "Jone's disease." It would be decades later and a world away before I realized the significance of that moment.

During World War II, at the age of 13, my father had been taken out of school to work on his own father's farm, freeing up older males for the military. He had no formal education, but between him and his ten brothers, all farmers, there was enough knowledge and support to make a living. My father's farm was our only sustenance, for which he worked tirelessly and with little reward. The dozen or so cows had to be milked twice a day, seven days a week, year-round. Herded into the two small cow byres—sheds, in America—the cows were tied to the stall with a chain around their necks, and the milking machine cups applied to their udders, one cow at a time, to extract a meager amount of milk. Pouring the results into a ten-gallon milk churn, the milk wagon would call daily, pick up the churns, and leave empty ones for the following morning. There were no vacations.

During breaks from medical school, I helped out when I could. I would help milk the cows and look forlornly into the churn and the few inches of milk in the bottom. This was a lot of effort for a miserable few gallons of milk.

A few years later, my father died young, from pancreatic cancer. He had made sure my sister and I had found a different career than farming. We took very little convincing. My mother went to live with my grandma in a local village, more serene than the farm, with central heating, hot water—the basics—while I emigrated to the United States, now a young surgeon. Navigating my way through the British and US surgical ranks was not always easy, but I knew I had brought the farm with me.

I just did not realize I had also brought the cow.

I was fortunate to work in some of the most prestigious hospitals and universities in Britain and the US: The University of Edinburgh, Royal Infirmary of Edinburgh, the Surgical Faculty at Yale University, and as a Colorectal Fellow at the Mayo Clinic, before finally entering private practice in Atlanta, Georgia. Missing academia and surgical research, I started a Colorectal Fellowship training program, the first in the state of Georgia. I am not even sure how it happened, or when it happened, but it gradually dawned on me that the dying cow, decades ago, did not die from "Jone's disease," but "Johne's disease." It was as if a light had just gone on in my head. "Jone's" was my father's Yorkshire interpretation of Albert Johne's (Figure 7), eponymous disease. In the years since, the connection between Johne's disease and Crohn's disease has fascinated me. Johne's disease in cattle is the equivalent of Crohn's disease in humans, and both, as mentioned earlier, are caused by a bacterium *Mycobacterium avium paratuberculosis*, or MAP.

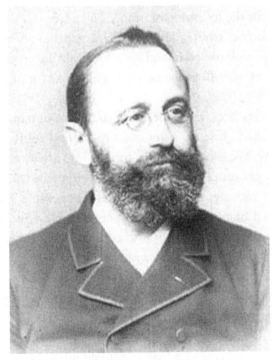

Figure 7. Heinrich Albert Johne. (1839-1910).

Over the years, I have developed a medication for Crohn's disease, which is now in clinical trials in Australia, Turkey, and Pakistan. (The US is too expensive, and Europe is too bureaucratic for clinical trials). Additionally, I created another treatment: a biologic "plug." It works by closing the holes (fistula) that Crohn's disease creates, and this treatment is now used throughout the world, from China to Chile. Since Johne's disease is a cattle disease, I formed a collaborative research program between myself and the Veterinary School of University in Athens, Georgia. Together, we as a team could hopefully detect and treat Johne's in man: Crohn's disease. After all, who better to detect MAP and Johne's disease than a veterinary surgeon?

The saying "you can take the boy out of the farm, but you can never take the farm out of the boy" is absolutely true. Imprinted with my father's toil, the endless days, and sleepless nights as a young surgeon were a little burden. A farm teaches self-reliance. If the cows have broken out of the field and are trotting down the rural roads, you grab your bike and chase after them, or they won't be back. If all the sheep follow each other (which they do, the saying is correct) over a break in the dry stone walls that checker the Yorkshire Dales, you rebuild it there and then, or they're also gone. If the tractor won't start because the battery is flat, as it always was, you run it down the hill for the farm, in first gear, clutch in, picking up speed toward the cliff edge at the end of the road. At the last minute, let go of the clutch, and the engine should fire into life. Just pray the brakes work, which, thankfully, they usually did.

Summer was hay-making season. We cut the grass with a tractor-mounted agricultural grass cutter, driving dozens of times around and around the pasture until it was all mown. Then, when the grass had dried after a few days, we'd do the same with the hay turner to expose the underside to dry. Then, when it rained, as it frequently did, repeat step #2 until the hays dry or dry enough. If it rained again, repeat again Then bale the hay, into 4x2 feet hay bales, stack all said bales into "stooks" of twelve bales. Then load all bales onto a trailer, drive to the hay barn, and unload all said bales. Hundreds of times. There were no Plan Bs. The cows needed to eat during the winter months when snow covered the fields.

In winter, the cows were kept inside the byres, away from the harsh winter. Straw, the leftover after harvesting wheat or barley, was used as bedding, sometimes fodder if there was no more hay left after a long winter. The land on our farm was too poor to grow barley, so we purchased fields of harvested corn, 20 miles away in the fertile Vale of York. The process was basically the same as making hay, but with an added 20-mile tractor and trailer drive through the local town, Ripon, and then back to the farm. The straw was baled, then stacked into stooks, in case it rained. As it frequently did. Arriving after school to help "stook" the straw bales, my heart sank as I gazed at hundreds of scattered bales strewn over the 25-acre straw field (roughly 25 football fields, the basic measure of all American life, as I was to find). We worked until it was pitch dark, our hands raw from lifting the baler twin and our knees bleeding from kneeing the brittle straw bales to the tops of the stooks. Driving a massive tractor, towing a 20-foot trailer stacked with ten courses of bales through the narrow streets of Ripon was a terrifying task. More than once, the load collapsed, spilling hundreds of straw bales into the country roads.

Compared to that, going 48 hours without sleep as a surgical resident was a cinch.

I learned improvisation. There are a million uses for baler twine, the hemp string that binds the bales together. Using an electric drill, it can be wound into rope to tie down the bales, pull tractors out of ditches, or deliver a calf trapped in the cow's pelvis.

Spring snowstorms were not uncommon on the moor, catastrophic timing for lambing season for the Wensleydale sheep. Late at night, my father would enter the house, a blizzard raging outside, carting one or two half-frozen, newly born lambs; their mother would have died at lambing. Dressed in his army-surplus heavy trench coat, tied by the ubiquitous baler twine, we would place them in cardboard boxes next to the blazing coal fire, the sole source of heat in the house. Rearing them by bottle feeding with cow's milk, the lambs would be an extended family, following us wherever we went.

If a less fortunate lamb freezes to death on the moor, from a freak spring snowstorm, the ewe is left with no lamb to suckle her precious milk. This was remedied by skinning the dead lamb and tying its little fleece (using baler twine) to another lamb whose mother had died during birth. The ewe would sniff the hide, and, believing it was her own lamb, would let down her life-saving milk.

To earn a little cash, I purchased a sow (female pig) and started breeding pigs. I discovered that pig muck was the most efficient decongestant in the world, its stench capable of permeating the most congested sinus. Each pig usually had ten or twelve piglets, who were born at surprising speed. Having slipped out of their mother's birth canal, the tiny, pink, hairless piglets would instinctively head to their mother's six pairs of teats for their first milk. Once the first six had claimed a nipple on the lower row, the next six would straddle their little brothers or sisters to reach the mother's second row of teats. This was the original "piggyback."

Lux et Veritas: "Light and Truth"

The farm was a million miles away from where I was going, but it prepared me well. Being a surgeon is no joke, and requires hours and hours of hard work, dedication, and determination. Two decades later, I was recruited to Yale University, whose university motto is *"Lux et Veritas"*—"Light and Truth." Finishing up a surgical residency and joining the Yale University faculty as a junior, attending, a certain amount of clinical research, publications, presentations, and lectures was expected. It was, after all Yale, home of Harvey Cushing and the spectacular Cushing Library, where I spent a great deal of my spare time. Teaching the surgical residents and eager young medical students, I provided some simple advice: when presenting a complex topic before a large audience, you have to repeat yourself to allow the audience to absorb the facts: "First, tell them what you're going to tell. Then tell them. Then tell them what you've just told them. Then they'll understand... if you're lucky." This has been a guiding principle during my thirty years' surgical career not only for myself, but for the near fifty surgical fellows in my colorectal surgical fellowship program.

As a practicing colorectal surgeon for thirty years, I certainly know Crohn's disease. Over the decades, I have operated on hundreds of Crohn's disease patients, who are ravaged by this mutilating disease. Many patients with Crohn's disease display similar characteristics, such as being young, impossibly wasted and bone-thin, chronic debility, and paleness of skin from blood loss. As if the physical toll isn't enough, Crohn's also plays a role in their relationships and socioeconomic status. Their families suffer with them, and relationships are strained, sometimes to the breaking point. Furthermore, these people often struggle to make ends meet, financially devastated from sky-high medical bills and mind-boggling expensive medications. Even the most dedicated and hardworking individuals fight a losing battle to keep a full-time job due to frequent hospital admissions. Most need surgery at some point. I have spent countless hours under the glaring OR lights, trying to dissect out the matted loops of bowel, struggling to figure out what is where and what needs to be removed and what can be saved . . . before the disease returns, as it usually does. These are the most difficult surgeries by far, not only because of the incredible inflammation it causes, or the torrential bleeding from friable, thinned blood vessels and the bowel, which is paper-thin and often disintegrates in your hands, but because not all survive. Infection after surgery, leaks from friable bowel, overwhelming sepsis, malnutrition, all can take their toll. Toby, a young patient of mine, immediately comes to mind. Although he survived and struggled through several abdominal surgeries, he was always bone-thin and in constant pain. Just as his body deteriorated from the inside out, his relationships slowly fragmented, and as a result, he was abandoned by his family. Alone in the world, he took his own life. He was tired of just surviving.

The role of MAP in Crohn's disease is a very complex subject. Toby, and others like him, fuel my passion to understand the role of MAP in Crohn's disease. To try and understand the deeply complex and controversial topic, I have returned to it hundreds of times, often in the early hours of the morning, as I lay awake shifting through data in my head, trying to sort the true from the false information. There's far too much false information circulating about the role of MAP in Crohn's disease, even in medical literature. These patients are deeply suffering; they deserve the best and absolutely to know and understand what wrecked their lives.

I have explored sources previously unknown to me. The weather patterns in Berlin in March 1882; the ship manifest of the British Royal Navy in 1721; *The New York Times* 1932 report of the Lübeck disaster; The German-English translation of Robert Koch's 1882 *Die Äetiologie der Tuberkulose*." I have read journals I would never have imagined—*The Journal of Environmental Epidemiology; The Journal of Veterinary Science; The Journal of Molecular Biology.* All to make the case.

To help convey the topic, I will take my own advice. First, I'll tell you what I'm going to tell you, then tell you, Then I'll tell you what I've just told you. Then you'll understand . . . if I'm lucky.

I have not been back to the farm since my father's death. I return frequently, but only on Google Earth. Amidst the lush green landscape of rural Yorkshire Dales, dotted with farms and villages, nestles a small, dilapidated farm on the edge of the Yorkshire Moors. There are no cows in the fields. An occasional white dot, a Wensleydale sheep, grazes the sparse grass. The wind and storms on aptly named "Hill Top Farm'" have stripped the galvanized sheets from the barn roof, many of the limestone walls have crumbled, and trees now grow in the pigsty, once the epicenter of my two-pig empire.

I always glance at a small stone cow byre, its slate roof long since collapsed, laying empty to the elements, where decades ago, a young boy stared at the wasted cow. He looked in dismay at her bowed head, sagged in silent despair. Her staring eyes sunk deep into their sockets, and her bare bones were protruding through her ulcerated, matted hide.

That was where this journey began.

CHAPTER 3

TOBY

It was just another Monday morning, the same as any other Monday for the past 25 years in my surgical practice. I greeted the nurses, sipped my hot chocolate, and sat down to sign prescriptions, review charts, and read report—just as I had for the past two and a half decades. I started to dig through the six-inch pile of charts, correspondence, and medical records. Two decades ago, the correspondence was typically run-of-the-mill, nothing too crazy. But as the years went by, it seemed to become increasingly more bizarre.

On this particular Monday morning, a disability request of six weeks was on my desk following a colonoscopy, a procedure which is performed under sedation, no incisions, takes 15–20 minutes, and the patient returns to work the following day. Although I admired this patient's creativity, it took unbelievable nerve, and it would never fly. Another first amongst many. Next, I picked up my annual scorecard from the hospital, which included lengths of stay, complications, deaths, and so forth. Basically, the school report for a surgeon. Only, we were compared to the surgeons that were the best of the best: Mayo Clinic's, the Cleveland Clinic's, Yale

University's. Overall, it looked like I was doing pretty well. Even though I typically operated on more complex patients with a more serious disease, on the whole, I had shorter lengths of stay, fewer readmissions, and, importantly, fewer mortalities compared to the average. *"Not too shabby if I do say so myself,"* I chuckled to myself. Next up was the infection control report card. After operating on a colon, in spite of using bowel prep and antibiotics, the occasional wound infection was inevitable. After all, the colon is home to billions of bacteria, and a couple of them are bound to escape even the most rigorous prevention procedures. But what to do when that happens? Standard protocol says to send the specimen to bacteriology. But I say, *"Don't."* If there is a wound infection, simply remove the staples, release the pus, and it will get better. If it is sent to bacteriology, it will inevitably create a report and be added to the scorecard with your name on it. This is not an inappropriate measure: it saves precious time and money. Besides, the treatment for localized wound infection is the same regardless, and as an added bonus, your wound infection rate miraculously disappears. My performance spoke for itself. If one looked at my infection rate on the graph compared to orthopedics, neurosurgery, OB/GYN, and ENT, my tiny little red bar was way on the left side of the bell curve. Far below anybody else's; incredibly below even neurosurgery, the most sterile of all procedures.

The next letter looked unfamiliar. Weirdly enough, the return address was a funeral home. Concerned and puzzled, I opened the letter, only to find a death certificate for Toby. Stunned, I sank back in my chair. Though I had not seen Toby in months, he had been a patient of mine for many years. He, like so many others, suffered from recurrent Crohn's disease. I had operated on him at least a half dozen times. Hurriedly, I scoured through the page looking for the cause of death—when I saw it.

Suicide.

I felt a wave of nausea pass over me. I almost threw up.
I thought back to how our journey had begun. When I first
met Toby, he was an impossibly thin 22-year-old kid. He had
had Crohn's disease for many years, lost a tremendous amount
of weight, was unable to eat or drink, had constant diarrhea,
and frequently was in pain. As a result of all the loops of matted bowel, he had a grapefruit-size, swollen mass in his right
lower quadrant, which had fused together due to the inflammation. Protruding from his shrunken abdominal wall, this mass
was visible even at a quick glance. Toby fell into the Catch-22
that is unfortunately all too common for patients with Crohn's.
With a chronic and incurable disease and suffering from constant pain, Toby was unable to work. Meaning, no income and
no resources. The only constant factor in his life was Crohn's
disease. Among several things, unemployment brings with it a
lack of health insurance. Although Obamacare covered many
conditions, not even Obamacare always covered such severe,
chronic conditions such as his. If available, the premiums for
Obamacare are frequently astronomically high. Tragically,
these typically young adolescents, unable to work and without
health insurance, are the most desperate individuals in society
that most desperately need health insurance.

Facing often multiple surgeries, costing unthinkable thousands
of dollars per admission, facing recurrence of his disease, Toby,
like many patients with Crohn's, had accumulated tens of thousands, often hundreds of thousands of dollars in unpaid medical
bills. Biologics, such as Remicade, Humira, Cimzia, and Stelara,
help suppress the symptoms of Crohn's disease, but they do not
cure it. They also cost tens of thousands of dollars per month,
impossible even for a highly successful individual to pay out of

pocket, far less an unemployed kid down on his luck. Toby was one in the legions of Crohn's sufferers.

When he needed another abdominal surgery, we developed a plan we called "the underground railway" to get him into the hospital without being confronted with an unpaid bill of hundreds of thousands of dollars. If patients end up in the emergency room, they are required to be treated in the same manner. Regardless of their insurance status, regardless of means, and regardless of outstanding hospital bills. The terms of the "COBRA" law mandate that any patient showing up at the emergency room is required to be treated in the same way as any other individual, whether they are insured, uninsured, able to pay, poor, broke, or homeless. The other alternative to get Toby into the hospital for another massive abdominal surgery would mean having him admitted as an "elective" case, registering in the hospital database, filling out reams of financial documents, and being confronted with an outstanding balance of tens of thousands of dollars up-front. But this is a terrible option. No uninsured person has this luxury. Toby did not even have a credit card. Accordingly, we used a tried-and-true route: the underground railway. This method had served us well during the many years of his illness. This underground railway was a scheme where he would show up in the emergency room whenever he needed abdominal surgery. He would bypass the demands of tens of thousands of dollars upfront and be treated like any other. Toby would then text me when he was in the emergency room, having registered as an urgent case, as he usually was, and I would show up, book the operating room, and we would perform the surgery. No demands for out-of-pocket money. With abdominal pain, his weight loss, and his diarrhea, Toby was going to end up in the emergency room sooner or later. This was not an abuse of the system; it was beating the system. If the system is so broken,

I was fine with abusing it anyways. The COBRA law is one of the greatest pillars of US health care, especially for treating uninsured Americans who have no good options. Certainly, the bills will arrive eventually, and the outstanding balance will stagger even further under its own weight. But at least patients are receiving treatment and care.

When I first met Toby, I surgically resected about 12 inches of intestine, the "grapefruit" in his abdominal wall. I managed to reconnect his intestines, a "re-anastomosis." Fortunately, we also avoided needing a stoma, "the bag," as patients not so affectionately refer to it. In the years afterward, his Crohn's disease was unremitting and relentless. Unable to afford any biological medications to suppress the disease, his Crohn's disease roared back with a vengeance. He experienced multiple recurrences over the years, each of them requiring resection of more and more bowel. Each of these surgeries was increasingly complex, with increasingly dense adhesions (scar tissue), more complex anatomy, increasingly severe bleeding, and less and less bowel left. After the third or fourth surgery in as many years, the only option for Toby was to create an ileostomy, where the bowel is brought to the abdominal wall and "the bag" is placed over it to collect the stool, which is emptied two-three times a day. Even then, Toby remained stick thin.

On his initial visit, he had a caring mother and a girlfriend of several years. Dad had disappeared years ago, when his Crohn's disease was first diagnosed. After the second or third admission, the girlfriend disappeared. After four or five admissions, Mum disappeared too. Toby was alone in the world. Even after five or six abdominal surgeries and a permanent ileostomy, Toby's life was not what the average 25-year-old would ever imagine for themselves. Tragically, even paying the near ultimate price of having a stoma, he developed a rare complication from his ileostomy where the Crohn's disease eats away the skin from around the stoma, called *pyoderma gangrenosum,* a hideous mass of inflamed, necrotic, bleeding, stinking tissue.

We relaunched our underground railway yet again. Toby rolled up in the ER at a designated time and day, got registered as an "urgent" case, and texted me. I arrived and scheduled his surgery. As an extension of the underground railway, and to book precious OR time, I would "schedule" a fake patient at a time that would work for us. When Toby needed surgery, I would call the OR scheduling staff, announce that "Patient X" had canceled, but I had another case to schedule in that same precious slot. It always worked seamlessly, and no one ever questioned the puzzling coincidence. Now, this was abusing the system!

I resected the diseased stoma and replaced his ileostomy from one side of his abdominal wall to the other, away from the pyoderma. Toby's abdominal wall was starting to look like a game of tic-tac-toe, with vertical, horizontal, and oblique incisions. But this was no game. He was now alone in the world. Abandoned first by his father, then his girlfriend, now by his own mother, Toby was left to fend for himself. After his most recent (and fatefully last) flare-up of the pyoderma, Toby could take it no longer, and took his own life. This would be a recurrent theme in the increasing tide of adolescents with Crohn's disease, and the story has tragically repeated itself time after time.

From Guns to Crohns

I did not always want to be a colorectal surgeon. Most medical students would laugh at the prospect. Unsure what I wanted to do, I entertained the prospect of being a spinal surgeon. During the final year of medical school, as students at the University of Manchester, we were allowed to take a three-month sabbatical to explore our careers, the profession, and the world. I landed a three-month sabbatical in Hong Kong, at the Duchess of Kent Spinal Orthopedic Hospital, which specialized in pediatric kyphosis and kyphoscoliosis.

This seemed like a reasonable, productive, and worthwhile career to follow. Spending three months in Hong Kong, operating on children with twisted spines, I soon realized this was not the specialty for me. The whole process seemed more akin to assembling kitchen cabinets, with screws, plates, bolts, and drills than surgery to me. Moving from Manchester to Edinburgh, the location of the Royal College of Surgeons, I started to plot my future surgical life.

Landing a prestigious residency job at Yale University, I was subsequently promoted to its faculty. I had more than my fair share of operating on gunshot wounds. Guns are illegal in England. The mantra in England is "have gun, go to jail." Not so in New Haven, Connecticut, on the fringe of the 1970's New York drug epidemic. Gunshot wounds rolled into the emergency room nose-to-tail, day and night, often multiple at any one time.

They were so common we were given instructions in self-preservation should an active shooter walk into the emergency room, which happened once or twice. On a 72-hour weekend call for surgery, the toll from operating on gunshot wounds was exhausting. Gunshot wounds are obviously less predictable than elective surgery, since the bullet can track anywhere through the abdomen, the vena cava ("Big Blue"), the aorta ("Big Red"), the bowel, or at random. After three days and nights of sleeplessness, constant surgery, and gunshot wounds, I received another call at 3:30 in the morning, having just laid my head down for ten minutes to grab some fleeting sleep. Another gunshot wound. "How refreshing," I murmured to myself as I pulled on my sneakers. I always slept in scrubs to avoid having to dress and trudged down to the emergency room. I soon realized, in my exhausted mind, I was walking slowly in the hopes that this next gunshot wound would possibly expire prior to my arriving at the emergency room. I soon realized that trauma surgery was not a good fit for me.

I elected to spend a further year in colorectal surgery. The colon is, after all, the largest organ in the body, so it seemed exciting to be able to do major surgeries and avoid the traumas and gunshot wounds. I landed a plum spot at Mayo Clinic in Rochester, Minnesota, and quickly grew my credentials as a future colorectal surgeon. Even at Mayo Clinic, which treated many famous politicians, Crohn's disease was interestingly rare. The runway of Rochester Municipal Airport was lined by 747 jets from Dubai, Kuwait, the United Arab Emirates, and many of the Middle Eastern countries, with people who came for the best of the best treatment, along with an entourage of friends, families, and many wives.

Crohn's disease was an oddity, even at this stage of my career. It was rare and seemed like something that only appeared in the surgical textbooks, rather than in real life. Twenty-five years later though, these roles have dramatically reversed.

Bright Lights

For a surgeon, the abdomen is divided into four quadrants: the right upper quadrant, home to the liver, the duodenum, the gallbladder, and the "hepatic" flexure of the colon; the left upper quadrant, land of the spleen; the right lower quadrant, where the cecum (first part of the colon) and appendix are; and the left lower quadrant, where the "sigmoid" colon twists down to the rectum. In the center of these quadrants, the small bowel twists and turns, absorbing nutrients and water. Sitting below all of these is the pelvis. Over the decades, I learned to be the most cautious in the right upper quadrant. It is the land of the largest veins that tear easily and gush torrents of blood, the most unpredictable anatomy, especially in Crohn's disease and dangerous monsters, the pancreas and duodenum, lurk in the darkness. This danger is enshrined in a favorite piece of advice which graduating surgical residents (trainees) deliver to the newly arrived neophytes, about to embark on their surgical training: "Eat when you can, sleep when you can, and stay away from the pancreas".

I have never lost a patient during abdominal surgery from bleeding, except for the occasional gunshot wound, which hit Big Red or Big Blue. But while operating on Crohn's disease, I have come very close to losing a patient from exsanguinating hemorrhage. It happens far too frequently.

Crohn's disease welds together adjacent loops of the bowel, which need to be untangled, and resected. Trying to free these up can result in massive bleeding from the dilated thin-walled veins that supply the bowel. This often results in massive bleeding, requiring two suctions in order to suck away the pouring blood. Sometimes the bleeding can be so ferocious, it makes a terrifying "swooshing" sound. The old surgical mantra is, "bleeding isn't bleeding until you can hear it." By then, you're in deep trouble. The mind races, the forehead sweats, the back tingles with goosebumps.

The left upper quadrant is not much of a problem. If the spleen starts to bleed, you simply mobilize it up, clamp its vascular supply, and remove it. The right upper quadrant can be terrifying, from the huge veins that drain the bowel into the liver. The most terrifying is the "confluence" of veins, second in size only to Big Blue. In Crohn's disease, these massive veins become paper-thin, and a tear can easily cause massive bleeding. Sometimes, the tear is impossible to find. Many times, I have packed a massive bleed, forcing huge pressure on the surgical pack with my clenched fist, and prayed. Sometimes the bleeding gets even worse with the pressure. Then you use two clenched fists and pray. There is a tense exchange between the surgeon and anesthetist, as they pour blood into the patient, trying to "catch up" with the blood loss. The scene is orchestrated by a rapid "beep beep beep" from the EKG machine, announcing the patient's slipping away. Blind clamping in deep holes is dangerous, but in this terrifying scenario, rapid, blind clamping is the last-ditch attempt to stop the torrents of blood. Thankfully, I have always managed to get a hold of the situation, and nobody has died "on table." It is a terrifying experience. Afterward, when the case is completed, I often experience a "postoperative high," akin to the man who has just dodged a bullet. Frequently drenched with sweat, a change of scrubs is often in order.

The pelvis and the lower quadrants equally are not as challenging when it comes to surgical bleeding. If the rectum in the pelvis is freed up from the sacrum, often thin-walled veins called the presacral veins, can bleed torrentially. These thin, friable veins can cause massive bleeding, again requiring two suctions to suction the literal tide of welling blood out of the pelvis. "The tide is coming in" is a frequent grim remark, black humor in an attempt to lighten the atmosphere in this terrifying scenario. The reason for this is these presacral veins are in direct connection with the inferior vena cava (Big Blue), which returns the entire recirculating blood supply from the lower abdomen back to the heart. If these presacral veins bleed, threatening an immediate exsanguinating hemorrhage, the simplest solution is to take a thumb tack from the poster board, sterilize it quickly, and press it into the bone of the sacrum, hopefully, to compress the responsible "pre-sacral vein," which, if properly placed, immediately stops the bleeding. I have known surgeons to carry a pre-sterilized thumbtack in a sterile "matchbox" around with them, ready in an instant, where the nurse can quickly grab it out of the surgeon's pocket. An inevitable sigh of relief ensues. With increasing regulation, these "right off the bulletin board" thumbtacks now must be purchased through an FDA-approved process to minimize the risk of nonexistent and imagined contamination. At hundreds of dollars apiece, these are very expensive thumbtacks.

Crohn's disease can create abscesses in the perianal region, which, when they burst, create a tract between the rectum and the outside of the perianal region, referred to as a fistula. These fistulas can be the most challenging problem in surgery. For years, the routine was to lay the fistula open, under anesthesia, and pack in this gaping incision for many months until it healed. This could result in bowel incontinence, incredible pain, and it was a mutilating wound, if it ever healed. I always encourage my colorectal fellows from my now near twenty-year-old Surgical Fellowship Program, to be creative and imaginative. I explain to them that if you are frustrated during a difficult procedure, make a mental note of the event and come up with a different, better, and simpler solution. This advice has proved immensely fruitful over the years.

For example, one day, it occurred to me that nobody had ever seen the inside of a fistula tract. My detractors scoffed at me though, saying, "Why would they?" In my own personal version of going to the dark side of the moon, I borrowed a very small diameter flexible scope, a ureteroscope, from the operating room. From there, I placed the scope into the fistula tract, and, for the first time ever, man saw the insides of a fistula. Even better, it all was caught on film. Thrilling, I know. I felt like I had just landed on the moon! I saw for the first time that the inner opening of the fistula tract was the key to fixing it. What it needed was a "plug." As always, my detractors were dismissive. But they still silently stared, gazing at the unfolding film. As excited as I was, these ureteroscopes are very fragile and prone to breaking, especially when doing a procedure they were never designed for. The urologists rebelled at their ureteroscopes being used, and seemed to be always "out for repair." Faced with a "urology coup," I was barred from performing my procedure. Storz, a German scope manufacturer, now makes custom-made "Fistulasopes," made especially and specifically for the job.

As a direct result of this "adventure," it soon became clear that the fistula "hole" on the inside of the rectum should be closed with a plug, rather than surgically laying the entire fistula tract open. Accordingly, I "requisitioned" a few small, postage-sized pieces of biological material, used for laying over the surface of the brain (a "Dural Patch") after brain surgery. Rolling one of these into the form of a golf tee, I gently inserted this new "Fistula Plug" pulled into the fistula "hole," so literally "plugging" the fistula. Stitching the plug in place, this closed the fistula tract without surgically laying it open. This avoided pain, incontinence, bleeding, and slow or non-healing of the tissue. After the first few patients returned to my office two weeks after surgery for a post-op check-up, I was delighted to find the fistula tracts had actually healed, more often than not, lifelong. This new invention, the "Biodesign Anal Fistula Plug" made by Cook Surgical in Bloomington, Indiana, created worldwide excitement and is used across the globe.

Further innovation resulted in new medication for anorectal Crohn's disease. As if mutilating the intestines wasn't enough, Crohn's can ravage the perianal area with deep, horrendously painful fissures (tears in the skin), deep fistulas, ulcers, and fleshy "elephant ears'" skin tags. When Crohn's localizes to the perianal region, the first line of treatment is an antibiotic, called metroni-dazole or Flagyl, which is taken by mouth to treat the anorectal region. But the Flagyl pills are very large, making them difficult to swallow. Not to mention the unpleasant, metallic taste. It always seemed ridiculous to me to have to use a nasty tasting pill by mouth to treat your backside. It seemed tantamount to putting toothpaste on your backside to clean your teeth. One morning, I had three patients in my office, each with devastating anorectal Crohn's disease, each of which had been on oral Flagyl for several weeks. All of them experienced a constant nauseous sensation and tingling and numbness in their fingers (peripheral neuropathy). Needless to say, all were very unhappy.

Out of desperation, I called the local compounding pharmacy in the local town and asked them to create (compound) the Flagyl as a topical cream, so I could have my patients use it, instead of the oral form to place on their bums. The results were spectacu-lar. Topical 10% metronidazole cleared up the anorectal Crohn's disease like snow in summer, and "Ortem cream" is now manu-factured by SLA Pharma in Leavesden, UK. Ortem is currently in Phase III clinical trials in Turkey, Australia, and Pakistan. In retrospect, this was an early indication of the potential important role of antibiotics in treating Crohn's disease.

PART TWO: THE ROAD TO CROHN'S

CHAPTER 4

BEAUTIFULLY BLUE

On a frozen midwinter morning of 1882 in Berlin, a gaunt, grey-bearded doctor peered down the eyepiece of his brass Carl-Zeiss microscope, a gift for his 29th birthday, a decade ago, from his wife Emma. The winter of 1882 was particularly harsh. The River Spree had been frozen for weeks, the first time in living memory. Berlin lay under a sheet of ice and snow, under a pall of smoke from the blazing wood and oil furnaces, making the rooms unusually warm, including those at the Kaiserliche Gesundheitsamt (Imperial Health Office). Retiring early in the freezing evening, the 39-year-old veteran researcher, Dr. Robert Koch (Figure 8), left his precious microscope slides in a neat pile among others on his cluttered laboratory bench to be examined in the morning. The glass slides, smeared with spit and tissue from tuberculosis victims and immersed in the researcher's signature blue dye, absorbed the unusual warmth of his laboratory. As the slides silently sat on the bench, the furnaces meanwhile roared overnight against the epic freeze. All the while, a minor miracle took place that night. Returning the following morning, he gently slid the coverslip under the 100x magnifying lens of his treasured microscope, a routine he had performed thousands of times in his ten-year career.

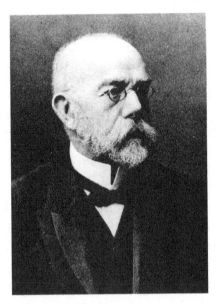

Figure 8. Robert Koch (1843-1910).

Robert Koch's blue eyes widened behind his gold-rimmed spectacles as he stared incredulously at what lay before him. Swarms of bacteria, "beautifully colored vivid blue rods, slender and tapering, clustered together in shoals," set against the brown background of its victim's dying phlegm. Their beauty belied their peril. For the first time in human history, Robert Koch had cornered and laid bare, in all their blue resplendence, the author of millions of deaths, pharaohs and emperors, Khans and czars, kings and queens, saints and sinners. The scourge of man and beast from the beginning. What lay before the eyes of Robert Koch, and the world, on that winter morning, was the tuberculosis (TB) bacteria, the killer of huge swathes of man and beast across the globe, since time began.

The History of Tuberculosis

During the population explosion in the Middle Ages, TB was rampant[37,38]. In the year 1882 alone, the year of Koch's discovery, TB was responsible for one-third of all deaths in his native country, Prussia. Unchecked, deaths from TB would globally translate to over a billion deaths per year in the 21st century. Its lesions were legion. In the crowded and unsanitary cities of Europe, TB was spread like wildfire from the hacking cough of its victims, creating a deadly aerosol which was duly inhaled by the next victim. But the real danger was found in its incubation time. The symptoms of tuberculosis often started years after the disease was revealed itself. So, an infected person could unknowingly infect other people for years before realizing the truth. As the disease spread from one person to the next, victims unknowingly swallowed the bacteria through their own saliva, and the bacteria proliferated in the intestine, causing abdominal cramps from narrowing of the bowel, loss of appetite, weight loss, intractable vomiting, and, finally, skeletal wasting. To "rest" the lung during the Middle Ages, the standard treatment was to insert a bayonet into the lung cavity and collapse the lung (pneumothorax). Thus deflated, the lung was expected to recover and gradually reflate over a period of weeks. Understandably, the technique fell into disrepute.

The church, seeing a huge potential revenue source, attributed the disease as an act of God on unworthy sinners, curable by papal salvation. In the Middle Ages, the disease was attributed to the "miasma" arising from the bowels of the earth. As mankind became more critical and analytic, they assumed that since the disease runs in families, it was therefore hereditary.

Tuberculosis, "the white plague'" of the world, had been ravaging mankind since ancient times. Its characteristic lesions have been identified in a fossil skull of Homo erectus, a half million years old, Egyptian predynastic mummies, and the skeletons of a 9,000-year-old Neolithic mother and child found in the Eastern Mediterranean. Tuberculosis was known to the Greeks and the Romans. Herodotus described the disease in his classic text *Histories.* Galen, Hippocrates Pliny the Younger, Aristotle all described the disease: *phthisis* (Greek), *consumptione* (Latin), *yaksma* (India), and *chaky oncay* (Incan), each of which makes reference to the "drying" or "consuming" effect of the illness: cachexia (wasting).

The often-quoted "romance" disease is hard to comprehend. British poet Lord Byron announced to the world, "I should like to die from consumption," helping to popularize the disease as the disease of artists. Certainly, compared to the "Black Death," (bubonic plague), the "White Death" (tuberculosis), was a more lingering affair. Young, fashionable women of the age blanched their complexions to mimic the romantic aura of tuberculosis. Many romantics, real and imagined, died in its grip. The mother of Edgar Alan Poe, Elizabeth, died at a young age from tuberculosis, leaving a distraught Edgar alone in the world. The icon of dark literature devoted his career to classics focusing on death, resurrection, and the afterlife. At the age of 26, he married his 13-year-old first cousin, Virginia Clemm, stating her age as 21 on their marriage certificate. The books became lighter, less bleak for a few years, such as *The Tell-Tale Heart* and *The Prose Romances,* until Virginia also died 11 years later at the age of 24, from tuberculosis. Another library of bleak literature followed—*The Raven* and *The Cask of Amontillado.* In October 1847, a disheveled, alcoholic, half-starved Edgar was found collapsed on a Baltimore street and died days later, likely from tuberculosis. In 1950, George Orwell, dying of tuberculosis, wrote one of his most famous novels, *1984,* and did not live to see it published.

The Bronte sisters, a literary powerhouse in Haworth, North Yorkshire, authors of the classics *Wuthering Heights* and *Jane Eyre,* all died from TB at a young age. Father to the six children, five girls, and one boy, Patrick Bronte, the vicar in Haworth, lived in relative affluence in the parsonage. The children were sent to "boarding school" for children of the clergy at Cowan Bridge. Here, the two older sisters, Maria and Elizabeth, died from TB whilst still in their teens. The one brother, Branwell, died in 1848 at age 31 from TB, but also apparently aided by a mixture of alcohol and opium. Emily, the author of *Wuthering Heights*, died from tuberculosis at the age of 30, just four months after Branwell. Anne, the youngest sister, died one year later, at the age of 29, before seeing her book, *The Tenet of Windfall Hall*, published. Charlotte lived long enough to pen *Jane Eyre*, a damning criticism of boarding schools. But she tragically died at the age of 38, from . . . guess again: tuberculosis.

The reason for the early demise of the entire Bronte family has recently been attributed to contaminated drinking water. The parsonage tapped its drinking water from a spring which was located in the same watershed as the Haworth Church graveyard, resting place of scores of TB-riddled corpses. Drinking the contaminated water for years has been proposed as the reason for the entire family's early demise, plus the close living conditions of all six children undoubtedly sealed their fate.

Presentations of Tuberculosis
Unlike many other diseases, tuberculosis has different presentations, depending on where it manifests in the human body. Scrofula, a disfiguring enlargement of the salivary glands and lymph nodes in the neck, starts as a localized infection in the lungs and eventually lodges in the lymph nodes and salivary glands through infected spit. On the other hand, Pott's disease targets the lumbar (lower back) vertebrae. More accurately, it

destroys the vertebrae. This gives the victim a twisted, painful spine and often results in a loss of their lower limb function, effectively crippling the victim as they await their inevitably slow death. Yet again, there is another form of tuberculosis described as intestinal TB. Intestinal TB often results in blockage of the bowel, agonizing cramps, diarrhea, and perforation. Like Pott's disease, people with intestinal tuberculosis often suffer an agonizing death. But the most common and contagious form of TB was, and still is, pulmonary (lung) TB. The classic symptoms of night sweats, drenching fatigue, a hacking cough, and spitting up blood (hemoptysis) are the classic signs of pulmonary TB. The initial focus in the lung, after inhaling the bacterium, starts as a primary lung nodule, the Ghon focus. Meanwhile, the disease continues to proliferate in the lung tissue, migrating to the apex of the lung, resulting often in large, cavernous spaces: bulla (Latin for spaces). Typically, the bullae expand to such a degree, they compress healthy lung tissue and condemn the victim to a slow, asphyxiating death. The unlucky victim dies a long, torturous death from wasting, shortness of breath, breathless asphyxiation, and continued hacking of blood from the infected lung abscess. A merciful end comes from a hacking, choking death from respiratory failure, as the body is consumed into a broken, skeletal contortion. Occasionally though, victims get lucky. And by lucky, I mean they don't die a long, agonizing death. Instead, the fortunate few are blessed with a quick and explosive death. In this case, victims would instead exsanguinate in his or her own lungs and rapidly drown in blood.

A normal, healthy small bowel (ileum) is the same diameter and general plasticity as a child's bicycle inner tube: a consistent, pliable, flexible tube of intestinal smooth muscle, propelling the intestinal contents down the bowel. Intestinal tuberculosis results in a rigid, fibrous, almost wooden narrowing of the bowel. The lymph nodes draining the diseased bowel become massively enlarged, to the size of marbles and even golf balls, filled with a cheesy material, known as caseous necrosis (Latin for cheese). The massively inflamed, entangled mass of bowel, mesentery, and lymph nodes forms a bloody, inflammatory mass that can often be felt through the abdominal wall as a painful, tender entanglement of bowel loops. The inability to absorb nutrients and the end result of complete bowel obstruction, a universally fatal condition until the early 20th century, resulted in a slow and agonizing death. It all ended in the final act of a grotesque play: consumption, the wasting, decaying, lingering end, with its night sweats and hacking blood. Tuberculosis was an invisible and prolific killer. Hardly anyone developed cancer in the 1800s. How could they? Everyone was dying from TB.

Koch Discovers Bacteria

Robert Koch[38,39], born in the silver-mining region of Clausthal, Prussia, now central Germany, the son of a mining engineer. The prodigy was the third of 13 children and taught himself to read and write at an early age. He entered medical school at the University of Gottingen and graduated in 1866. The subsequent year, he married Emma, and the two had a daughter, Gertrude, the following year.

Koch was no newcomer to tracking killers. In 1878, volunteering as a surgeon in the Franco-Prussia War, he had ample opportunity to study septicemia, gangrene, and cellulitis in the wounded Prussian soldiers. Way ahead of his time, he studied, isolated, stained, and even photographed the responsible bacteria, displaying them for the world to see for the first time ever. Germany was home to a massive dye industry, a byproduct of its huge oil imports from its African colonies, Ostafike (East Africa), Sudostafrika (Southwest Africa), and central Africa. Hence, Germany had access to a wide variety of materials. Using the vast array of newly available dyes, Koch experimented with combinations of colors, different staining sequences, immersion times, alcohol and alkali washes, and potassium hydroxide fixatives. Some of his favorite dyes were aniline blue, methylene blue, fuchsia red, and vesuvin (Bismarck brown). Ironically, he used the same fabric dyes to color the uniforms of the Prussian soldiers sent to war in the Franco-Prussian War: red for the infantry, red and brown for the artillery, and deep red for the cavalry. The Prussian army was certainly the most colorful army, but the French regiments had the Prussians beat in style and flamboyance. Unfortunately, fashion was the only thing in which the French beat the Germans. Coming in a very poor second, the Franco-Prussian war lasted only a year. The French forces were routed, Paris occupied, Alcase-Lorraine annexed by Germany, and the French with a five-billion-franc war reparations bill.

During Koch's early life, the prevailing theory was the disease was caused by "internal vibrations" within the victim's flesh. This was the explanation for maggots eating decaying flesh, flies emerging from dead tissue, and gangrene consuming a wounded soldier. Only a few outliers proposed the disease was from "foreign parasitic cultures." Koch believed that diseases were caused by external bacteria, and that there were different and distinct species, rather than each morphing from a common progenitor. He also believed that each bacterium produced its own specific disease, and these diseases could be reproduced by injecting the responsible bacterium. Benjamin Martin, in 1720, suggested that consumption was caused by "wonderfully minute living creatures" and transmitted by "contagious living fluid." He went on to explain very likely that by a "habitual lying in the same bed with a consumptive patient, constantly eating and drinking with him, or by very frequently conversing so nearly as to draw in part of the breath he omits from the lungs, a consumption may be caused by a sound person. I imagine this likely conversing with consumptive patients is seldom or never sufficient to catch the disease." Martin's theory of "little animals" was ignored for 100 years.

Using the methyl violet dye, Koch isolated bacteria from the battlefield wounds of the Prussian army and was the first to not only identify, but also stain and culture the bacteria. Inadvertently, he almost single-handedly developed the process of microbiology and microscopy. Rigging the newly developed Eastman Silver bromide dry plate camera to the eyepiece of his treasured Zeiss microscope, he took the first microphotographs of the elusive microscopic pathogens, creating a brand-new technique of photomicroscopy.

In 1878, seven years after the Franco-Prussian War, Koch reported his experiments on the causes of several types of wound infection, such as abscess, gangrene septicemia, and cellulitis. He then reproduced these infections by inoculating animals and reproducing the original specific type. He successfully identified, stained, and photographed each bacterium responsible for killing wounded Prussian soldiers, on and off the battlefield. On the battlefield, gram-positive cocci streptococcus resulted in gas gangrene septicemia and cellulitis, which led to a mercifully quick death. But off the field, soldiers suffered a long and lingering death from purulent, discharging abscesses and putrefying wounds from staphylococcus-filled wounds. Discharged from the Franco-Prussian War and promoted to the University of Berlin, on Kaiserswerther Strasse, Koch now turned his gaze and his Carl Zeiss microscope to the tubercle bacillus.

Tuberculosis: Cause of "The White Death" is Discovered

On a fateful evening, Koch left the microscopic slide containing the sputum of a patient with consumption sitting in a solution of methylene blue, pending the following day's experiments. Unbeknown to Koch, the unusual heat of the room caused the tuberculosis bacilli to soak up the alanine dye during the prolonged exposure. The following morning, Koch resumed his experiment, picked up the discarded slide, washed it with a counterstain of vesuvin, and slid it under the 100-times viewing lens of his treasured microscope. Koch stared in astonishment at the vivid bright blue rod laying before him and his microscope. The tuberculosis bacteria for the first time in history lay before the eyes of Robert Koch, and the world. Koch subsequently described his bacilli as "beautifully blue, striking, vivid blue" and "in size and shape they bear a striking similarity to leprosy bacilli. They have been differentiated from the latter as being a bit slenderer and by having tapered ends." Leaving the microscopy slide sitting overnight in the warm methylene blue, Robert Koch had accidentally identified the tuberculosis bacterium for the first time in history[39].

Unknown to Koch, the tuberculosis bacterium possessed a thick and waxy coat of glycolic acid, the reason why it had resisted all prior staining methods. A similar scenario would be attempting to stain a candle with ink. The dye simply runs off the waxy coat, leaving no trace of its presence. Twenty years later, Lowenstein would finesse Koch's technique to include immersion with methylene blue, heating the slide, fixing with alkali, and counterstaining with vesuvin. In addition, Lowenstein added the clinching step of adding acid to the preparation to bleach off the dye from all by-standing bacteria, leaving them invisible under the microscope. Because the TB bacillus resisted bleaching by acid bath, it was given the name "Acid Fast Bacteria." Many more family members would be discovered in the decades to come.

Weeks later, on the evening of Friday, March 24, 1882, he presented his findings to the monthly gathering of the Physiology Society of Berlin. His lecture, "The Etiology of Tuberculosis"[40], was a world-changing event. Almost 10,000 words long, it was delivered before a stunned audience. Koch started his lecture with a reminder to the audience of the toll which tuberculosis had laid on mankind: "If the number of victims which a disease claims is the measure of its significance, then all diseases, particularly the most dreaded infectious diseases, such as bubonic plague, Asiatic cholera, etc., must rank far behind tuberculosis. Statistics teach that one-seventh of all human beings die of tuberculosis, and that, if one considers only the productive middle-age groups, tuberculosis carries away one-third and often more of these." Not a great orator, frequently adding uns and urs between sentences, Robert Koch's delivery took over an hour. The audience, shocked and stunned, sat motionless. There was no applause. No murmurs. No discussions. Only silence.

Bringing along his slides, specimens, reagents, and photographs for all to see, Koch laid bare all of the evidence he possessed. Intrigued, the dozen or so participants rapidly crowded around to see the evidence firsthand. Paul Ehrlich, a young dermatologist attending the lecture, recounted this was the most "important day in his professional career." He ran back to his home to reproduce and confirm Koch's findings. Years later, Ehrlich would produce the first treatment for syphilis.

His publication[41], "*Die Aetiologie der Tuberculose,*" or in English, "The Etiology of Tuberculosis," was published in the *Berliner Klinische Wochenschrift*, on April 10, 17 days later, sending shockwaves across the world. After a rapid translation, it was published in England in *The Times* on April 22, and in the US in *The New York Times* on May 3, 1882. Robert Koch was now a famous scientist and later became known as "The Father of Bacteriology[41]."

Attempting to culture tuberculosis was proving as difficult as it was to stain. Unlike anthrax, tuberculosis failed to grow on the conventional culture mediums of the day. Not even the ox's eye was helpful in growing tuberculosis, which was so successful for the anthrax cultures. Only when Koch extracted serum from the blood of sheep and cattle, and warmed it repeatedly to form a semisolid medium, did the tuberculosis bacterium grow.

Not only a fastidious eater, the bacterium, required a very specific and very narrow temperature range, never before encountered. Anthrax bacteria would grow anywhere from 34 to 40 degrees. The TB bacillus demanded a narrow range of 37 to 38 degrees of incubation: any lower or higher, the bacterium lay dormant. Without these exacting preconditions and prerequisites, the prima donna of bacteria refused to grow or proliferate.

The tuberculosis bacterium was a picky eater. Even then, the cultures took weeks to reveal themselves as flaky colonies on the agar medium. Half filling test tubes with his serum, and tilting them at an angle to increase the surface area, Koch inoculated the surface of the semisolid medium with the tuberculosis bacterium. A colleague, Petri, noticing his colleague's difficulties with his "tilted test tubes," suggested using shallow circular dishes with lids to prevent outside contamination. The petri dish is still the standard means of bacterial culture in modern times

Even after the bacteria were coaxed into multiplying, the cultures took weeks to reveal themselves as flaky, waxy colonies on the serum culture medium. Koch inoculated the surface of the semisolid medium with the tuberculosis bacterium. Using a flamed platinum rod, Koch sampled a tiny sample of the colony and transferred it to a fresh culture medium, sub-culturing the bacteria to obtain an ever-purer strain of the bacillus. After repeated transfers, he obtained an increasingly pure strain of his bacterium and set the stage to identify subcultures of a hitherto unknown strain of his bacillus

But Robert Koch was not finished. Having isolated, stained, photographed, and propagated the bacteria, he now moved on to demonstrate how the bacteria were transmitted. By injecting samples of this single bacterium into the abdomen of guinea pigs, rabbits, cats, monkeys, and cattle, Koch thoroughly tested how the microorganisms could travel from one species to the next. He examined transmission from apes to guinea pigs; cattle and monkeys to guinea pigs; humans to rabbits; monkeys to rabbits; monkeys to cats; and humans to dogs. Robert Koch left no stone unturned. The only permeation Robert Koch did not describe was experimental animal-to-human or human-to-human transmission, obviously due to the lack of volunteers.

By transferring samples from Koch's original cultures to subsequent generations of pure cultures, further strains of mycobacterium were subsequently isolated. For example, Mycobacterium Bovis is a close cousin to TB and is found primarily in cattle. However, it lacks the virulence of the human tuberculosis bacteria. Moreover, Mycobacterium avium was also discovered; this strain is endemic in birds. A close cousin to the Mycobacterium family, Mycobacterium avium would soon loom large in the hunt for Crohn's disease.

In Koch's hunt for the killers of the 19th century, and with his experience in isolating, purifying, transmitting, and replicating bacterial diseases, he defined his four Koch principles for defining a bacterial cause of infectious diseases: First, the organism must always be present, in every case of the disease. Second, the organism must be isolated from a host afflicted by the disease and grown in pure culture. Third, samples of the organism taken from pure culture must cause the same disease when inoculated into a healthy, susceptible animal in the laboratory, and fourth, the organism must be isolated from the inoculated animal and must be identified as the same original organism first isolated from the originally diseased host. The four Koch principles are a mainstay in the eradication of infectious diseases to this day.

Unfortunately, Koch went one step too far. In an attempt to treat the disease, he developed an extract of pure, attenuated tuberculosis bacteria, and injected it in the arms of victims in the hopes of producing a cure. Instead, these patients developed a massive reaction at the injection site, with fevers, collapse, and several deaths. Furthermore, the site of injection became necrotic with massive tissue loss. With the failure of his "Tuberculin" treatment to produce a cure for consumption, Koch's reputation dwindled. The Prussian state voided his patents for the treatment, and public opinion turned against the icon.

Although he failed to produce a cure, other scientists discovered that a diluted form of the treatment could test for immunity to TB, the tuberculin test. When performing the test, a small amount of the tuberculin extract is injected beneath the skin. A red welt at the injection site denotes immunity to TB, leaving a permanent scar. Despite the tuberculin disaster, Robert Koch received the Nobel Prize a quarter-century later for his work on tuberculosis.

An effective antibiotic, streptomycin was not available for another 45 years after first identifying the pathogen. The elusive tuberculosis bacterium was at first susceptible to the new antibiotic, but very shortly became resistant. New therapies required two, then three combined antibiotics. The tuberculosis bacterium was proving as difficult to kill as it was to catch

Paul Ehrlich, who was present at Koch's presentation, reasoned that the bacteria which were stained by the toxic dyes may also kill the organisms, leading to a potential cure. Coining his premise as a "magic bullet" against bacteria, Paul Ehrlich was absolutely correct, and his crazy theory is the mainstay of many modern antibiotics. Years later, Ehrlich would develop the first antibiotic against the other plague of the 18th century—syphilis. In March 1890, he developed a hacking cough, coughing up blood-tinged phlegm. He placed a specimen of his phlegm on a microscope slide, immersed with methylene blue, heating the slide, fixing with alkali, and counterstaining with vesuvin, adding acid to the preparation to bleach off the dye. Peering down his microscope Ehrlich's heart sank on seeing bacteria "beautifully blue, striking, vivid blue," "in size and shape they bear a striking similarity to leprosy bacilli." Paul Ehrlich had TB.

CHAPTER 5

DISASTER

In 1908, the Department of Commerce and Labor published the results of the first USA census. Although only 17 northeastern states, including California and Colorado, participated and the entire South did not, the 133-page document gave the first, largest, and most detailed mortality data of any nation in history. Classified by age, sex, color (white, Negro, or Indian), location, time of year, and occupation, the census data was revealing. At 78,289 deaths, the most common cause was, by far, tuberculosis, followed by pneumonia at 51,811. Far down the list was cancer at 22,214.

That same year, Albert Calmette, a French bacteriologist, and his assistant Camille Guerin, a veterinarian, were developing a culture medium for tuberculosis at the Institut Pasteur de Lille in Lille, France. The methodology involved experimenting with various culture mediums to grow and propagate the tuberculosis bacterium, including agar plates, egg medium, the favorite ox bile, and potatoes. Various combinations of each culture medium were tried, but the combination of the glycerin-potato-ox bile mixture seemed to inhibit the growth of bacteria the most compared to the agar and egg mediums.

Painstakingly, Calmette and Guerin took samples from each culture medium and transferred them to a new medium to isolate a purer substrain of the bacillus. To do this, they used a small, thin metal rod with a metal loop at one end to scoop out tiny samples of culture medium and bacteria and transfer them to a new culture medium. Thinking ahead, the pair smeared the samples in four or five quadrants to increase the surface area for growth. But between each transfer of bacteria, it was essential that the loop be placed in the flame of a Bunsen burner in order to kill any bacteria that were on the loop. Failure to observe this simple practice would result in cross-contamination from one sample to another, rendering the whole process futile. Today, we have plastic disposable devices which are disposed of between each individual use thereby bypassing the need to "flame" the loop, and hence avoid errors. In 1908, no such disposable culture loops were available. After repeating the subculture multiple times, Calmette and Guerin noticed that with each subsequent subculture, the bacteria became weaker and weaker, thus producing an attenuated strain.

Attempting to reproduce Jenner's smallpox vaccine experiment, the pair religiously sub-cultured the attenuated bacteria multiple times. By doing this, they hoped to further reduce the bacterium's virulence and create a live culture that would be suitable as a vaccine. But they noticed a drawback. They realized the colonies growing on the glycerin potato mixture often clumped, making identification of individual colonies less accurate and harder to loop individually.

To address this problem, they added diluted ox bile to the medium, which acted as a detergent, dissipating the colonies around the surface of the mixture. This spread the colonies out. Once the individual colonies were clearly distinct, creating subcultures became much easier and more reliable. Using the glycerin-bile-potato mixture, the pair sub-cultured the bacteria every three weeks. Subculture after subculture after subculture. After each passage, the virulence of the bacteria was tested on experimental guinea pigs. If the guinea pigs died, the bacterium was still virulent and unsuitable for human vaccination. But if the guinea pigs lived, they had reached their goal of a safe, non-virulent vaccine, suitable for human use. The process continued through World War I, even after the German's overran Lille. Determined to not let even a war get in the way, the pair sub-cultured the bacteria a total of 239 times in 13 years until they were confident they had sub-cultured a pure, attenuated live vaccine.

But disaster struck. Under German occupation, potato prices suddenly escalated because of the thousands of hungry German soldiers that now occupied the country. Then to make matters worse, the supply of ox bile came to a tumbling halt. Because the German army sequestered the entire cattle supply in northern France, ox bile was suddenly extremely difficult to obtain, not to mention the surge in price. But respite came in the form of the Lille Garrison commander. He was aware of the Koch Institute in Germany and his pre-war collaboration with the Institut Pasteur in Paris, and he, therefore, arranged for supplies of ox bile to be collected and delivered. This act of wartime benevolence clearly saved the decade's old experiment from failure and ensured that the vaccine would be available for widespread use in post-war Europe. Calmette and Guerin transferred to the Institut Pasteur in Paris after the war in 1919, and their vaccine was finally considered safe for human use two years later, in 1921.

But the vaccine was met by a skeptical public. Initially, its use was limited to infants born to mothers who were dying or died after childbirth from tuberculosis. The chance that these infants would succumb to tuberculosis was extraordinarily high, and it was felt that the vaccine would be not only their best, but only hope of survival. Samples of the tuberculosis vaccine now called the BCG vaccine were sent from the Institut Pasteur in Paris to various centers around Europe and the world. On July 27, 1929, a strain of BCG was sent from the Institut Pasteur to Dr. Altstadt in Lübeck, Germany, who passed the vaccine on to Professor Deycke at the General Hospital of Lübeck. Once the vaccine was received, it was inoculated into animals to ensure that the strain was not virulent. Samples of the same vaccine were sent to Mexico and to Riga, Latvia, and these centers used the vaccine on 3,016 infants without incident. This important fact will be critical in the disaster which was about to unfold in Lübeck.

Prior to administration of the vaccine, Calmette and Guerin made sure to keep the BCG strain on a medium of glycerin-bilateral leg-potato before transferring it to a liquid medium. Dr. Deycke, however, transferred the vaccine culture into an egg medium, which is a more potent medium. Meaning, it increased the bacterium's virulence. It is unknown whether he added the essential element of hematin, the cofactor required for tuberculosis growth. When Dr. Deycke's lab prepared the vaccine, BCG was taken from the egg nutrient agar and transferred to a glycerol glucose solution, where the desired concentration of bacteria was measured and titrated. Each vaccine dose, amounting to 2 cc was taken from the resulting mix and delivered to high-risk children of consumptive mothers. Each child would receive three doses of the vaccine within the first ten days of life, each dose separated by three days. Ideally, each child would therefore receive a total of 6 cc of the BCG vaccine orally.

A Tragic Blunder

By tragic coincidence, Deycke's lab also experimented with live TB[44]. Prior to receiving the BCG vaccine from the Institut Pasteur,

Deycke had several cultures of live tuberculosis bacteria, but due to an accidental rise in the temperature of the incubator, these cultures were killed. However, in September 1929, Deycke received a further shipment of live tuberculosis cultures from Kiel. This strain was originally isolated in 1927 from a child with tuberculosis of the hip at the Charite Hospital in Berlin. The following year, the culture was handed to the Robert Koch Institute and labeled H-29. In April 1929, a sample of the H-29 live bacterium was forwarded to the Hygienic Institute at Kiel, where Dr. Deycke's laboratory obtained its new sample. Dr. Deycke kept the live bacteria in an incubator in a large room and it was sub-cultured only on a fluid medium. As a comparison, when the BCG strain arrived from Paris in April of that year, five months earlier, it was kept in an incubator in a small room in the laboratory and was sub-cultured on the standard glycerin-bile-potato medium. The lab tech responsible for taking care of both the live bacteria from Kiel (H-29) and the BCG vaccine was an assistant who had been with Dr. Deycke for 17 years.

On December 9, 1929, Dr. Deycke was ready for his first innoculations[45]. Three high-risk infants were immediately brought forward. The first child had been removed from birth from his mother, who was suffering from open tuberculosis. A second child was vaccinated three weeks later, on December 30, 1929. Six weeks later, a third child underwent vaccination. Over the subsequent weeks, all three children developed signs of tuberculosis. The first child developed cervical lymphadenitis (swelling of the lymph nodes in the neck) which Dr. Deycke attributed to contamination of the child during delivery through the birth canal of his consumptive mother. To determine if the lymph nodes were actually infected with tuberculosis, Dr. Deycke inoculated a sample of the lymph node into a guinea pig, which died from generalized tuberculosis. The second child developed a positive tuberculin reaction, and the third child developed mild symptoms of tuberculosis. Unfortunately, all three died.

Undaunted, Dr. Deycke continued his program of immunization in full force. The main vaccination series commenced two weeks later, on February 24, 1930. Over the course of the next two months, 251 high-risk infants, about half of the children born in the Lübeck Hospital, were inoculated with the usual three doses at days three, six, and nine of life. By April 17, six weeks after the vaccination program had commenced, a child vaccinated 33 days previously died, presumably from tuberculosis. The mother denied an autopsy. Three days later, a second child died. The autopsy: generalized tuberculosis. Since the lesions were most markedly in the lungs, Dr. Deycke again concluded that the child had been contaminated from his mother's body fluids, which doubtless were rife with live bacteria. Over the next five days, two more children died. There were just too many dead babies. At this point, Dr. Deycke, realizing the deaths were due to the vaccine, abruptly halted his vaccination program and critically destroyed all the remaining vaccines in the lab. This step was carefully scrutinized in the subsequent investigation[46].

A public inquiry[47] was initiated, headed by Professor Ludwig Lange of the Reich Health Office and Professor Bruno Lange of the Robert Koch Institute in Berlin. The results of the subsequent proceedings were under national and international scrutiny. Of the 251 children inoculated, 72 had died by the following spring. Sixty-two children remained alive, but severely ill, 94 slightly ill and 17 children were apparently alive and well, although tested positive for TB. A small number of children died of unrelated causes. According to Dr. Klotz, director of the Children's Hospital in Lübeck, the children suffered from swelling of the cervical glands, often the size of hen's eggs, which caused an obstruction of the airways. And frequently, death. The children typically developed severe anemia, high intermittent fever, prolonged vomiting, profuse diarrhea, and emaciation. In the children who underwent autopsy, the typical hallmarks of intestinal tuberculosis were found—strictures of the gut, perforations, and massive lymph node enlargement within the abdomen. Each of these organs was teeming with live tubercular bacteria.

The remaining samples of H-29 and BCG were sent out to midwives and escaped Dr. Deycke's purging. After these samples were examined, many of them were found to contain virulent tubercular bacilli. More importantly, the strains resembled that of the killed sample—H-29. Two conflicting theories rapidly evolved. One group accused Dr. Deycke and his laboratory of inadvertently contaminating the BCG with the live H-29 virus and inoculating the children. Chief among these was the Institut Pasteur in Paris, who had supplied the original BCG vaccine. One strong line of evidence was the fact that samples from the same batch as supplied to Lübeck had also been supplied to Mexico and to Riga. There, a total of 3,016 children had been inoculated without any adverse outcome. Therefore, it appeared that the BCG vaccine sent to Lübeck had been non-virulent and safe to use as a vaccine. The other group had a very different idea about what happened. Opposing this theory were the supporters of Dr. Deycke who were, understandably, in the minority. These individuals claimed the BCG samples sent to several centers around Europe and the world had been analyzed and live bacteria had been cultured. Their main line of evidence was that the attenuated bacteria spontaneously became virulent over a period of time, making the whole concept of BCG vaccination both dangerous and immediately life-threatening. But there was another piece of evidence on the table.

This one lay in the timing of the inoculation of the children and their subsequent deaths. The resulting inquiry focused less on how the contamination had occurred, but more on how the children had died. The average time from inoculation to death in all 72 infants was 42 days. Some infants, however, survived longer, up to three months or more.

So, the investigators then turned to the midwives and nurses involved with the administration of the tuberculosis inoculant. Subsequent deposition proved the process was very flawed and inconsistent. For example, many lucky infants either vomited some or all of the TB inoculants or developed severe diarrhea, both of which eliminated the potentially deadly bacteria from their bodies. This revelation led the investigators to another piece of evidence. They carefully and meticulously analyzed the timing of the infant deaths and realized the mortality rate varied depending on when the vaccine was distributed. For example, vaccines sent out in the last week of February and the first four days of March had the highest mortality rate. In fact, this particular batch led to the highest mortality in all 72 victims. Interestingly enough, after this, there was a quiescent period of ten days in which comparatively few deaths occurred, despite some infants taking all three doses. And the pattern continued. Following that, there was a short period of three days when the vaccine again caused a very high proportion of death. Finally, during the last two weeks of the vaccination program, the bacteria appeared to be non-virulent. In retrospect, the timing of administration of the vaccine and the deaths pointed to the source of contamination: mixing of the H-29 and BCG samples. This provided a lethal inoculation.

In hindsight, the most likely source for this was the simple inoculation loop used to transfer the colonies from culture to culture. A failure to perform the crucial sterilization of the loop may have caused cross-contamination of the fatal H-29 tuberculous bacteria into the BCG vaccine.

The Lübeck Trial[46], held in the Lübeck Town Hall, lasted for three months. Reaching its conclusion on July 4, 1932, Dr. Deycke was sentenced to 18 months in prison and his assistant to two years.

The disaster and its aftermath came with an unlikely twist[48]. The judge in the trial was admitted to an insane asylum with a diagnosis of "melancholic insanity," but was released a few weeks later, apparently cured. He checked into a small hotel in Hamburg and committed suicide by shooting himself in the head with a pistol. The reason for his suicide was said to be because the convicted doctors had planned to appeal their verdict on account of his insanity.

CHAPTER 6
THE CURSED FIELDS

Albeit 21 years his senior, the paranoid and reclusive Louis Pasteur (Figure 9) was a contemporary of Robert Koch. Born in 1822 in Dole, France, Pasteur was a lifelong French Nationalist, which would make him a natural antagonist to Koch, and result in academic conflict later in their careers. The son of a soldier, Pasteur began life with humble beginnings and gravitated toward the arts in his early life. Painting pictures of his friends and family, Pasteur eked out a meager living. One of his favorite art forms, lithography, would prove invaluable in his future years in the unlikely sequence of events that would result in a new method of food decontamination, named pasteurization, after its creator.

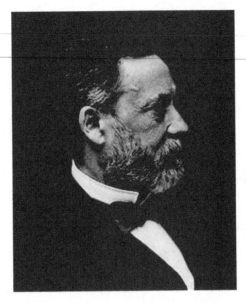

Figure 9. Louis Pasteur. (1822-1895).

Lithography involves the transfer of an image on a solid wood or stone surface and transferring that image by contact printing to a parchment or paper reproduction. The two images thus formed are mirror images of each other, and this concept of mirror images of objects, otherwise known chemically as isomers, would prove critical in cracking problems with fermentation. The process began a whole new discipline of chemistry known as stoichiochemistry. The two images created in lithography, as when an object is held up to the mirror, are identical but mirror images of each other. If you look at your hands, you'll find a similar analogy. Your right and left hands are strictly identical, but opposite copies of each other. Mirror images are known as chimeras, the Latin word for hand. In the world of chemistry, they are often referred to as isomers.

Pasteur evolved from the world of art to pursue a career in chemistry at the École Normale Supérieure. His early work involved research of the crystalline compound tartaric acid and lactate. One day, Pasteur noticed that if a light were transmitted through a solution of lactate, it would consistently rotate polarized light to the left. Curious, he set out to discover why this happened. Eventually, he discovered that the isomers found in nature, including organic solutions such as tartaric acid, were almost exclusively levo-isomers, which can be metabolized and made by living things. When transmitting light through a solution, he discovered that counterclockwise rotation produced levo-isomers and right-sided rotation dextro-isomers. The opposite of levo-isomers, dextro-isomers cannot be created naturally or developed metabolically in nature. Instead, they have to be manufactured chemically in a laboratory by a chemical reaction or by heating, but never by a natural process.

Excessive heating of wine produced a compound known as para tartaric acid, which has an identical molecular structure, melting point, and physical properties as its native tartaric acid; however, para tartaric acid failed to rotate polarized light. The inquisitive Pasteur refused to believe the conventional wisdom that these two compounds, tartaric and para tartaric acid were identical. Being the meticulous and obsessive person that he was, Pasteur examined crystals of para tartaric acid under a microscope and, using a pair of tweezers, separated what he recognized as two mirror images of this same molecule. Had it not been for his background in lithography, this excruciatingly minute detail would almost certainly have been missed.

After separating the two crystal isomers of tartaric acid under a microscope, he created two tiny piles of the individual crystals and dissolved them in solution. When he shone polarized light in the tartaric acid solution, the light deviated to the left but deviated to the right in the para tartaric solution. And when the two solutions were mixed, there was no deviation of light in either direction. Based on this last piece of data, he rationalized that each crystal counteracted the effect of the other. Such a solution of equal portions of two isomers, both levo- and dextro-isomers, are referred to as a racemic mixture.

Pasteur had created the new discipline of stoichiochemistry. This was not just a quirky chemistry experiment: Stoichiochemistry would be pivotal in the most devastating medical disaster in history, over a century later: The Thalidomide tragedy.

Thalidomide

In 1956, a German chemical company, Chemie-Grunenthal, joined the search for an effective antibiotic against tuberculosis, headed by Dr. Wilheim Kunz. The resulting medication would become to be known as thalidomide. As an antibiotic, thalidomide was useless; however, Dr. Kunz noticed that all of the experimental animals were asleep in their cages. The new "wonder drug" was marketed as a sedative and hypnotic, and by 1957, 47 pharmaceutical companies were marketing thalidomide in as many countries.

The Distillers Company, a British pharmaceutical company, licensed the new drug and distributed the medication under the brand name Distaval in Britain, Australia, and New Zealand. In 1960, the Distillers Company rep in Sydney approached Dr. David McBride, a high-profile obstetrician, suggesting he prescribe the new medication for morning sickness. Anxious to try anything new to maintain his reputation, Dr. McBride handed out the medication to his pregnant patients. Months after, in the spring of 1961, Dr. McBride's midwife, Sister Sparrow, was shocked when she delivered a child with horrific limb deformities. The arms, the forearms, and lower limbs were absent, and vestigial hands and feet were protruding from their shoulders and hip joints, a horrific deformity, termed phocomelia. A shocked Sister Sparrow had never seen the like of this in her life. Two weeks later, she delivered two more infants with the same hideous malformations.

Sister Sparrow was quick to identify the underlying cause-Dr. McBride's new thalidomide medication. Initially dismissing her claims, Dr. McBride quickly acquiesced as several more children were born with the same mutilating deformity. Dr. McBride wrote a brief, five-sentence letter to *The Lancet*, describing the possible association between thalidomide and phocomelia, ending his inquiry "Have any of your readers seen similar abnormalities in babies delivered of women who have taken this drug during pregnancy?" Around the world, similar malformations had also been seen and Dr. McBride became an international hero, receiving multiple accolades including a cash award from the L-Institut de La Vie in France. Unfortunately, in the four years that thalidomide was dispensed to the public, approximately 10,000 newborns were afflicted by this horrendous malformation, and many more thousands died from cardiac and visceral malformations.

Many years later it became apparent that thalidomide existed in 2 forms, which Pasteur had described 100 years previously. The mirror image of these two stereochemical forms of the medication was present in every thalidomide pill. The mirror images, the "R" form (dextra) was therapeutically effective and produced sedation and alleviated morning sickness. The other isomer, the "S" form, (levo) was not only ineffective, but resulted in embryonic limb deformities.

The drug was rapidly removed from the market and doctors were instructed to destroy any supplies of the medication they possessed. Fortunately for the US, the medication was never authorized by the FDA for use in North America. This near tragedy led to a dramatic re-vamping of FDA requirements for drug research and development, one which still, fortunately, remains in force today.

Pasteurization

Back to Pasteur. Transferring at an early age of 25 to a Paris École Normale in Strasbourg, Pasteur met the daughter of the dean of the university and subsequently married the same month. Of the five children that were born to the couple, three died of natural causes, further concentrating Pasteur's determination to know the secrets of mother nature.

Later, Martin Strasbourg, a local brewer, approached Pasteur to investigate a recurring problem in his beetroot beer mix, which frequently produced sour beer rather than the sweet alcohol-laden product. And it wasn't just him. This problem was brewing across the nation, becoming a national emergency. Direct communication from Napoleon III resulted in Pasteur taking on the project, recruiting his local students, and visiting the breweries in southeast France. Together, they realized the sour taste was due to an accumulation of lactic acid, which produces the same sour taste as in sour milk.

Turning again to his crystal theories, Pasteur dissolved a sample of the souring compound into a solution of water. Passing polarized light through the solution resulted in the characteristic left-sided shift: the one produced by living organisms. Being sure that the reason for the spoiled vintage was due to an organic organism, Pasteur further examined samples of sweet alcohol-laden beer and the soured samples. In the sweet alcohol-laden samples, Pasteur saw plump, healthy yeast cells. In the soured batch, the yeast cells were much smaller, fewer, and interspersed with multiple rod-like bacteria, which Pasteur correctly indicated was the source of the souring.

Before Pasteur's discoveries, fermentation was thought to be due to "internal vibrations," which were intrinsic in grape solutions and caused the breakdown of sugar in the grape juice to produce alcohol. Additionally, it was thought that these vibrations could be transferred between vats of wine. Running contrary to popular belief, Pasteur announced his findings that the souring was due to these small, rod-like bacteria. Not internal vibrations. Convinced that the yeast was the source of the fermentation process, Pasteur removed samples from the interior of the grape, thus avoiding the yeast cells located on the grapevine on the skin of the grape. Attempting to ferment the interior of the grape, by excluding the fungi, resulted in no fermentation process. Adding back the grape skins with the yeast returned the fermentation process to its normal state. Pasteur even collected samples of air from various altitudes, including sea level and up to high altitudes in the French Alps, in order to determine if these yeast cells were present in the air. Sure enough, the air collected from sea level and low altitudes resulted in a normal fermentation process, and the high-altitude air devoid of yeast resulted in no fermentation. To clinch the argument, Pasteur developed his famous swan-neck experiment, making a flask with a curved or swan neck. Grape juice was added to the interior of the flask and was boiled to 60 degrees Celsius, then the tip of the neck was sealed to exclude contaminants such as dust and yeast. But the solution failed to ferment. When the tip of the glass was broken at its tip, leaving the U-shaped flask, again no fermentation occurred. But when the neck was broken close to the flask, air, dust, and the contained yeast cells entered the interior of the flask and it resulted in fermentation. Pasteur, therefore, disproved the theory of spontaneous vibrations and demonstrated the process of fermentation was due to yeast cells carried in the air. To state it another way, the process of fermentation was a biological process due to living organisms. In this case, yeast.

Pasteur went on to further elaborate his process of pasteurization and discovered other benefits to boiling fermented liquids to 60 degrees Celsius. In addition to killing potentially contaminating bacteria, boiling liquids also limits the production of lactate, which maximizes the production of alcohol—an essential in the wine industry. A typical concentration of alcohol rose to 10%–15%, whereupon the yeast cells became inactivated. The process of pasteurization would not evolve to its use in milk for several decades. This delay would result in many thousands of tuberculosis deaths in European children drinking contaminated milk.

A Lucky Break

Following on from his works in pasteurization, Pasteur turned his attention to chicken cholera. After reading Jenner's studies on inoculation of smallpox, he concluded a similar process may be possible for chicken cholera, then endemic in rural France. He received live cultures of chicken cholera from Toussaint and cultivated them in chicken broth. In 1878, Pasteur hired Charles Chamberland to assist him in this new project. Immediately, the pair embarked upon serial culturing of chicken cholera, administering them to chickens and observing their rapid demise. Unbeknownst to Pasteur, Chamberland was disinclined to work. But this, inadvertently, was a blessing in disguise.

In 1879, Pasteur left for a rare vacation. He instructed Chamberland to inoculate yet a further batch of chickens with the virulent cholera. Rather than perform his appointed tasks, the idle Chamberland also left on vacation, unbeknown to his master. Returning a month later, he found the spoiled culture sitting on the benchtop with a dark and opaque color. Rushing to cover his blunder, Chamberland quickly inoculated a batch of chickens, expecting them to die. Surprisingly, the chickens survived and showed no sign of disease.

In a rare moment of introspection, Chamberland meekly approached Pasteur with this news, assuming the batch was spoiled and useless thanks to his idleness. Pasteur, however, instructed Chamberland to infect the chickens with a live cholera vaccine. Expecting the chickens to die, Pasteur realized spoiled culture broth may actually prevent the disease in chickens. The pair repeated the experiments with the spoiled culture in a further batch of chickens and injected a second batch with a live vaccine. Again, the batch injected was spoiled, the culture survived the inoculation with a virulent chicken cholera vaccine, but those injected with fresh virulent cholera culture died rapidly. Were it not for Chamberland's idleness, this important discovery would have gone unnoticed. Presenting his findings to the French Academy of Sciences, Pasteur concluded that that the original virulent culture had become attenuated or weakened by exposure with air, thus spoiling or attenuating the culture.

Intrigued by his discovery, Pasteur set out to see if his immunization methods worked on other diseases. Having heard about Robert Koch's studies on anthrax, Pasteur turned to anthrax and got to work. Rural France was peppered with outbreaks of anthrax in "cursed fields," where cattle died routinely and were buried in the same field. Pasteur suspected that the disease was being brought to the surface from the buried cattle by earthworms and moles. If that were true, the buried cattle could therefore be a source of the recurrent infestation in these fields. Excited by this prospect, he meticulously studied earthworm excrement (likely one of the few to be excited by worm poop). Just as he thought, he found the bacteria in earthworm excrement, demonstrating that this was a plausible theory. Pasteur theorized that exposure of the anthrax bacterium to air, like the chicken cholera, could weaken the bacteria, and therefore make it a potential vaccine. Injecting the air-exposed anthrax vaccine, however, routinely killed cattle. Clearly, the oxygen method was not working. Meanwhile, Pasteur's arch-enemy, Henri Toussaint, suggested using the powerful oxidant carbolic acid (potassium dichromate), recently described by Joseph Lister to kill the bacteria, then injecting them into sheep and cattle. Pasteur dismissed this and insisted that his oxygen method was correct. Unbeknownst to everyone else though, Pasteur had stolen the idea of using potassium dichromate as an oxidizing agent from Toussaint and would use the vaccine in front of a skeptical public. The famous French veterinarian, Dr. Hippolyte Rossignol proposed that a live experiment be performed to test Pasteur's vaccine under the careful scrutiny of the French Academy of Science. Pasteur accepted the challenge, and the famous experiment was scheduled at Pouilly-le-Fort, using otherwise healthy cows, sheep, and goats.

The experiments at Pouilly-le-Fort started on May 5. A total of 31 animals were immunized: six cows, one goat, and 24 sheep. Twelve days later, they received a follow-up vaccine on May 17. As a control group to compare to, 29 animals were left unvaccinated: four cows, one goat, and 24 sheep. The day of judgment was set on June 2, 1881.

Two weeks later, in front of a growing crowd, Pasteur and his three assistants injected live anthrax cultures into the inoculated animals. Many of the onlookers were skeptics and joined the crowd to witness Pasteur's greatest failure. But when the morning broke and Pasteur arrived, he was greeted by applause and cheers by the onlookers. At two o'clock in the afternoon, the tally was counted. All of the 24 vaccinated sheep were alive and well, compared to 21 of the unvaccinated sheep, which were lying dead in the field. Of the few remaining unvaccinated sheep, they were clearly sick, and all three were dead by the end of the day, two of them dropping dead in front of the audience and spectators. Gazing quizzically at the excited crowd, the six vaccinated cows were healthy and grazing quite happily in front of the audience. The four unvaccinated cows were clearly sick, swollen, feverish, and near to death. Pasteur had gambled his reputation and possibly his livelihood by this live experiment, risking public humiliation and disgust.

Fortunately for Pasteur, the experiment was an unequivocal success. The reclusive and paranoid Pasteur, however, failed to disclose that he further attenuated the spores with potassium dichromate, similar to how Toussaint had proposed carbolic acid. Not wishing to share his findings with his colleagues, Pasteur committed his findings to his notebook, which he donated to his son after his death with instructions never to publish.

On to Rabies

A few years later, Pasteur turned his attention to treating and preventing rabies, then endemic in both rural and urban France. A bite from a rabid dog carried a mortality of anywhere between 5%–60%, depending on the extent of the bite, bite depth, and tissue damage. In December of 1884, Pasteur began injecting strains of rabies virus into the brains of experimental rabbits. After the virus had incubated for two weeks, he then harvested the spinal cords from the rabbits, cutting them into strips to be dried. To speed up the attenuation process, Pasteur used potash to dry the air. The strips were then pummeled into a liquid and left to be exposed to air for varying periods of time: 12, 13, or 14 days. After the exposure time was complete, the liquids were then injected into the spinal columns of 50 rabid dogs.

According to Pasteur, his experiment on the 50 dogs had been an unparalleled success, and none of the dogs infected with rabies died. In July, nine-year-old Joseph Meister arrived from Alsace with his mother, having been bitten by a rabid dog two days earlier, on July 4. The dog had been killed by its owner, who accompanied Joseph and his mother to visit Pasteur. On July 6, Joseph and his mother arrived at Pasteur's door, begging to be treated. In December of the previous year, he had turned down a child under similar circumstances, fearing his vaccine was not yet perfected, resulting in the child's death from rabies. But now, Pasteur felt he was justified in starting this experimental treatment. Having gained reassurance from two local physicians, including Dr. Roux, Pasteur realized that the young Joseph would otherwise be "doomed to inevitable death." With Dr. Roux in attendance, Pasteur started the series of injections that same evening. Starting first with the strip that had been drying for two weeks, the first injection was in Joseph's abdominal wall, followed by 12 more injections over the course of the following ten days, using an increasingly virulent vaccine, which had been dried for shorter periods of time, culminating in the last day with only a one-day-old vaccine preparation.

To Pasteur's understandable delight, young Joseph survived the series of inoculations and showed no evidence of rabies. Initially, there was cause for concern. A week earlier, Pasteur also had treated a second boy, 15-year-old John Baptiste Jupille, who had been attacked by a rabid dog while defending his sheep herd. But John Baptiste arrived at Pasteur's laboratory six days after the attack, compared with two days for Meister. Tragically, the boy died. Pasteur had already risked prosecution by treating John, especially as a non-member of the medical profession. To lose two boys within weeks of each other could have instantly ruined his career. So, when young Joseph recovered, Pasteur was relieved. Three months later, when Joseph Meister was examined, he was found to be in good health. Over the course of the following year, Pasteur inoculated a total of 350 people, including children from around the world and the United States.

Adapting his immunization regimen to account for the fact that John Baptiste's disease was likely more advanced than young Joseph's, Pasteur escalated the vaccine schedule. Young Jupille, like Joseph, survived the vaccination regimen, showing no signs of clinical rabies. A week earlier, the ten-year-old Louis Pelletier, who had been bitten 37 days prior to arriving at Pasteur's laboratory, was less fortunate. Having firmly established itself in the central nervous system of Louis, the virus ultimately took its toll, and he, unfortunately, passed away. Driven by this loss, Pasteur knew he had to take his vaccine a step further: injecting it into healthy individuals. It wasn't enough to only treat sick people; he had to also prevent them from catching rabies. So Pasteur then took the final, risky step of injecting his vaccine into unaffected individuals, as a precaution against a potential rabies bite. This further extension of his vaccine drew criticism and skepticism from the medical establishment. In spite of this, the Institut Pasteur was established in Paris in 1886. The institute became a magnet for patients from all over Europe seeking his preventive treatment. By the time of his death, Pasteur had vaccinated a total of 20,000 individuals from all over the world, with a mortality of less than 0.5%. In 1931, 51,057 people had been treated at the Institut Pasteur in Paris, with only 151 deaths, a mortality of 0.3%.

By sheer guesswork, common sense, and a dash of good luck, Pasteur took the first steps in determining the proper dosage, duration, and frequency for vaccines. Not only that, but he also realized that an escalating vaccination program was more suitable for heavily infected and high-risk individuals. These principles hold true even today.

Battle of the Laureates

The conflict between Koch and Pasteur developed early and intensified as their respective careers and fame evolved. The contributors were geopolitical, professional rivalry, and mutual distrust. The background to this was the Franco-Prussian War, which was a conflict engineered by the German kaiser, Otto von Bismarck, with the intention of uniting the disparate German state. Lasting only two years, the conflict resulted in complete humiliation of the French military and the capture of Emperor Napoleon III at the Battle of Sedan. Due to greater German efficiency, overwhelming numbers, and French ineptitude, the conflict culminated in the siege of Paris and the decimation of the French armies.

The surrender terms included a five-billion-franc reparation to be paid by the French to the victorious Germans and the annexation of the provinces of Alsace and Lorraine. Louis Pasteur, a professor at the University of Strasbourg in the annexed province of Alsace, had a good reason to hold a grudge against Germany and the nationalist German Koch. In addition, his only son, Jean Baptiste Pasteur, was a soldier in the French military during the Franco-Prussian War. The French and Germans were also in a geopolitical chess game, along with Great Britain, to colonize the various tropical African states, which would require an intense program of immunization against tropical diseases like cholera, typhoid, and malaria.

Pasteur's legendary secrecy and deception in relation to his scientific reporting, findings, and experiments were a constant undertone to the German Koch. Pasteur and his increasing litany of followers believed that bacteria could be weakened or attenuated by various methods. When his chicken cholera had become weakened by exposure to air, he falsely claimed that the anthrax vaccine had been weakened by exposure to oxygen before stealing his colleague's method. Koch had discovered the powerful oxidizing agent: potassium dichromate.

Not only did Pasteur steal Jean Joseph Henri Toussaint's method of attenuating the anthrax bacteria using potassium dichromate, but he attacked the idea as ridiculous, unworkable, and ineffective. Secretly stealing Toussaint's method of attenuating the anthrax bacteria, and following his public experiments in the French countryside, Toussaint's reputation was in ruins. He died shortly after from a "nervous condition," widely thought to be the result of his ruined career. Tensions flared after Pasteur's successful vaccination of the child Meister with his rabies vaccine. Fortunately, his experiment was successful; however, at the time, only 50% of bites inflicted by rabid animals resulted in the full clinical syndrome of rabies, with photophobia, drooling, seizures, and, ultimately, death. Pasteur may have been fortunate, but Meister may not even have developed the disease, although he claimed credit for saving his life. Pasteur's career was also focused on self-enrichment and propagating his reputation through a series of Pasteur institutes.

His publications about his vaccines (chicken cholera, anthrax, and rabies) were intentionally short, lacking detail, and misleading. Pasteur never failed to file patents to protect his ideas and to cash in on his discoveries. At one point, Pasteur and the Institut Pasteur received no less than 10% of the total financial grants provided by the French government.

The US. embraced the German Koch to the detriment of Pasteur. The dean of American Medicine, William Welch, director of the Rockefeller Institute for Medical Research and first president of the newly formed Johns Hopkins University, traveled to

Germany to study Koch's methods and to bring them back to the US. Having established the first public health school at Johns Hopkins Hospital introducing Koch's methods to America, Welch soon disavowed Koch as World War I approached.

As a result of America entering World War I against Germany, the United States confiscated the US patents and trademarks developed by Koch and the newly formed German companies, Bayer, AG, and Merck. Koch's reputation soured as a result of World War I, and Pasteur took the opportunity to propagate his reputation at the opening of various Pasteur institutes in Paris, Europe, and even China.

Although Pasteur was claimed as a national hero after his death in 1895, he committed his documents to his family, insisting on their secrecy. In 1964, his last surviving male descendent, Pasteur Vallery-Radot donated 106 laboratory notebooks to the Bibliothèque nationale de France. Kept under lock and key for over 150 years from prying eyes, the notebooks were released to researchers. Once this happened, Louis Pasteur's darker side became public. Dr. Gerald L. Geison of Princeton University examined each of the 106 laboratory notebooks, written in a tiny, meticulous hand, and found gaping discrepancies between Pasteur's personal notes compared to his public, published claims.

Pasteur's use of Toussaint's potassium dichromate technique at Pouilly-le-fort was revealed. The second flagrant departure between Pasteur's stated method, and his secret method was during the vaccination of the French child with the rabies virus. Pasteur claimed he had successfully used the vaccine in 50 dogs. This was not the case.

Faced with his first patient, Pasteur departed sharply from what had been successful in his alleged dog experiments. Pasteur embarked on a dangerous series of injections into the young boy at daily intervals, using vaccines that became more potent with every daily injection. This untried rapid escalation of virulent bacteria greatly increased the child's exposure to the rabies virus. Fortunately for Pasteur, either the child had not contracted the sufficient viral load to cause the flagrant symptoms of rabies in the first place, or his instincts for using an escalating dose regimen was a lucky guess.

After all, Pasteur was a chemist and not a doctor. Over the years, he had accumulated enough enemies who were ready to pounce at any unsuccessful attempts. The full disclosure of Pasteur's deception was published in the *New York Times* by Lawrence K. Kaplan[43] on May 16, 1995, titled "Revisionist History Sees Pasteur as Liar Who Stole Rivals Ideas." The article made for disturbing but fascinating reading and an insight into the darker side of a scientist who played fast and loose with the rules, destroyed his friends and competitors with equal alacrity, and committed the real truth to his relatives to be locked up for over a century before the truth was aired.

CHAPTER 7

THE MILKMAID

An Unlikely Ally Against Crohn's Disease: Smallpox
In the last two decades, an unlikely ally has emerged in the fight against Crohn's disease: the deadly smallpox. The weakened pox virus was developed by the Jenner Institute at the University of Oxford and Professor Hermon Taylor as a vaccine against Crohn's disease. The deadly virulent virus was attenuated (weakened) by transferring it hundreds of times through specific culture media, just as TB was attenuated by Calmette and Guerin. Once the virus has been sufficiently weakened, it is no longer capable of dividing and multiplying in the recipient's body, avoiding a complete outbreak of smallpox. Thus, the once lethal virus transforms into a reliable, benign, "Trojan Horse" to carry Crohn's disease antigens inside the cells of the immune system (macrophages). The macrophages then coordinate the production of immune T-cells, which become sensitized to MAP. This destroys them, providing a viable treatment for Crohn's disease. Although in its very early stages, the idea is the vaccine may be used to treat Crohn's disease, as well as prevent it. Unfortunately, the first pivotal trial in Crohn's patients was put on hold because of the Covid-19 pandemic.

In a bizarre coincidence, the initial pox virus was developed in Ankara, capital of modern-day Turkey, part of the historic "Levant." Named the "Modified Vaccinia virus Ankara" of "MVA," the virus was initially inoculated into the hides of goats or donkeys, to develop an initial stockpile of the still deadly virus. Ironically, the initial vaccinations against smallpox were also developed in the 1700s in Constantinople (modern-day Istanbul), the capital of the Ottoman Empire. The Levitan method involved injecting pus from the sore of a smallpox victim under the skin of the healthy recipient, thereby inducing an immune response and lasting immunity from the disease. Obviously, this technique was very crude. Understandably so, disasters were commonplace, but immunity was assured.

History of Smallpox
Smallpox has a deadly track record through the millennia. The earliest records describe a disease that closely resembles smallpox in China around 4000 BC. Later, its footprint can be found in ancient Egypt, dating back to the predynastic Egyptian era from 3000 BC based on a smallpox-like rash found on three mummies from that era. The mummified head of Ramses V, who died in 1156 BC, shows evidence of smallpox. The disease then spread south down the Nile, emerging in Africa, eastward across the Ottoman Empire, and across the Mediterranean to Europe.

Smallpox first arose in Europe between the 5th and 7th centuries and has been implicated in the fall of the Roman Empire, where the plague of Antonine in 108 AD accounted for almost seven million deaths. Originally described as "variola" by Bishop Marius of Avenches in Switzerland in AD 570, the virus thrived in the most densely concentrated, overcrowded, and unsanitary

European cities. Unwilling to relinquish its death grip on European cities, the disease ravaged the citizens, and millions died.

Later introduced into South America in 1521 by Cortez, the disease then wiped out up to 90% of the indigenous Aztec population. Unknown in the new world, the conquistadors brought smallpox from Spain and Portugal and infested the local Aztec populations, which they decimated and subjugated for the next 300 years. Next, smallpox made its appearance in America. Shortly after the first settlement, Jamestown in 1607, the virus quickly spread between the settlers, which also likely caused the settlers' disappearance. Some malicious settlers even deliberately transmitted the deadly contagion to indigenous local tribes by gifting smallpox-infected blankets, thereby eliminating the vast majority of hostile Indians. By 1633, the Mohawk tribe was practically nonexistent, soon followed by the Iroquois in 1679. By 1770, smallpox had depopulated the plains' Indians. One colonizing Puritan wrote: "The good hand of God favored our beginnings in sweeping away the multitudes of the Natives by the smallpox."

The American colonists, being unfamiliar with the European plagues such as the Black Death, regarded the newly introduced plague in sheer horror. The medical historian Patricia Watson described smallpox as "the sudden and terrifying scourge" for American colonists. Boston, one of the largest centers of urbanization in the 13 colonies, was the focus of repeated smallpox epidemics, recurring every 12 years. In the much larger expanses of rural America, the disease was almost unknown. During epidemics, especially in Boston with its packed population, the "Speckled Monster" resulted in mortality rates up to 50% in adults and 80% in children. The sudden onset of this new disease, its unpredictability, and signs and symptoms like pain and disfiguration created horror in the colonies. The historian, Donald R. Hopkins, explained the true horror of smallpox was due to "the sudden-ness and unpredictability of its attack, the grotesque torture of its victims, the brutality of its lethal and disfiguring outcome, and the terror that it inspired." Smallpox was unique amongst human diseases.

Symptoms of Smallpox

Wherever smallpox struck, the pattern was the same: after an incubation period of 12 to 14 days, the victim erupted with sudden chills, fevers, backache, nausea, vomiting, and hallucinations. Following an outbreak of sores in the mouth, throat, and nose, an explosion of poxes appeared, first on the chest, back, torso, and face, before spreading outward (centrifugal) to the feet, palms, legs, and hands. This characteristic outward spread of the rash contrasted with smallpox's less virulent cousin, chickenpox. Chickenpox typically started on the arms and legs before spreading centrally (centripetal) to the trunk, chest, and abdomen. The fevers, disorientation, and raking muscle and back pain of small-pox typically lasted six to eight weeks, as the pox marks aggregated often, creating huge blistering masses with the characteristic sweet smell. The acute disease often resulted in blindness, osteomyelitis, and a prolonged death from encephalitis and respiratory failure. If the victim survived, there was a scabbing of the acute skin lesions, which progressed deep into the skin, causing mutilating ulcers on the face, arms, legs and torso, leaving a permanent record of the disease. Gradually, if the individual survived, the scabs fell off during the last weeks of the disease, resulting in a permanent "pox-marked" skin. This conveyed a permanent record of the patient's infection and a lasting guarantee of immunity against future infections from smallpox, including that of George Washington, who contracted the disease at the age of 19 in Barbados.

Immunization

The practice of inoculation had been practiced as far away as in China. In the 6th century, the Chinese took scrapings of the pox pustules, dried them to a powder, and had the patient sniff the powder into their nostrils, in a very early, but very practical form of inoculation. Since smallpox was and is primarily an airborne illness, transmitted to the mouth and the nostrils would not only be sensible, but very likely an effective means of immunization.

In West Africa, the practice was to inoculate through an incision in the arm, leading to a shortened attenuated form of the disease. The practice of immunization against smallpox, known as variolation, spread eastward through the Levant and the Ottoman Empire. There, the technique was refined, and its use disseminated throughout Europe and across the Atlantic to the American colonies.

In 1714, Emmanuel Timoni, physician and son of the interpreter at the sultan's court in Constantinople, refined the process of variolation. Having the distinct advantage of being multilingual, like his father, and medical training at Oxford and Padua, Timoni published the first medical description of the technique in the 1714 issue of *Philosophical Transactions of the Royal Society* in London. Fluent in English, Latin, Greek, and Turkish, he was able to convey this knowledge to England, Europe, and the American colonies.

The Levant practice was to collect pus from an active smallpox pustule, into an almond half shell. The pus "lymph" was then injected via a large needle into a vein of the patient's choosing, usually at four or more locations on the body. The injection sites were then covered with almond shells to ensure the inoculum was not wiped away. The immunizations were usually performed by "elderly Greek women," who were practiced in the technique. Patients were typically scheduled after the summer heat had abated, such as September or October.

The practice was crude and haphazard, and, in England, the new treatment was initially denounced as un-English and harmful. However, early experience with the method in Europe showed some promising results. Once inoculated, the recipients were immune from smallpox. But it also carried a significant mortality rate of up to 10% in otherwise healthy and uninfected individuals, including the two youngest sons of George III: Princes Octavius and Alfred. In 1722 the physician William Wagstaffe, it was a method totally strange to English constitutions, imported from "an illiterate and unthinking People" living in a warm climate, but "on a spare Diet, and in the lowest manner, almost without the common Necessaries of Life".

In 1715, the English beauty and socialite, Lady Montagu, contracted the disease in London, and, although she survived, her face was permanently mutilated with deep, disfiguring pocks. But smallpox was no new face to her. Her brother had already died of the disease a few years earlier. A year after her run-in with smallpox, Lady Montagu accompanied her husband, the newly appointed ambassador to the Ottoman Empire, to Constantinople, where she witnessed the practice of variolation first hand in the Ottoman court. Soon afterward, a smallpox epidemic hit Constantinople. Desperate to save the life of her five-year-old son Edward, Lady Montagu summoned the Embassy physician, Dr. Charles Maitland, with instructions to have Edward inoculated in the Levant manner. The elderly Greek women were summarily ordered to carry out the procedure, and young Edward survived the experience and did not contract smallpox. Returning to London a few years later, Maitland was again summoned, and Lady Montagu ordered him to inoculate her four-year-old daughter, who likewise survived the experience. To confirm the safety of variolation to a skeptical England, Maitland performed the procedure on six prisoners in Newgate Prison, in return for a royal pardon as well as several orphans of the City. All six prisoners and the orphans survived the experiment, and the practice was validated. As the recognized authority of variolation, Charles Maitland was appointed physician to the Royal Court, and soon performed the procedure on the two daughters of the Princess of Wales in 1722.

But the processes of inoculation were no new feat to the Indians and Negros in America. In fact, they had been practicing the art for years, albeit in a trial-and-error method. The Christian colonists regarded this as a heathen practice and interference with God's plan for humanity. As one clergyman quoted, smallpox was "a judgment of God sent to punish us and humble us for our sins." Because of this, many Puritans banned the practice of inoculation. But others saw the benefits and voiced their opinions. Slowly, more and more American citizens became receptive to the idea of inoculation.

But despite its early success, this very crude method inevitably met with the occasional disaster. If too much contaminant was introduced into a healthy recipient, the victim could develop a fully-fledged case of smallpox. Or even death. Worse still, a contaminated case could potentially propagate to other unvaccinated individuals, creating a minor epidemic.

HMS Seahorse

In 1721, Boston was one of only three dense population centers in America (along with New York and Philadelphia). Because of this, it was also the epicenter of disease. In the past five decades, the city had already experienced six major smallpox epidemics. Interestingly enough, each epidemic returned every 10–15 years like clockwork. In the years 1649, 1665, 1678, 1690, and 1702, smallpox spread among the inhabitants of Boston "with great destruction in life." In 1702, the worst to date, 313 persons died under its power. By 1721, Boston was almost 20 years overdue for its next smallpox epidemic. The population had long lost immunity from the disease, and Boston's herd immunity had dwindled. Herd immunity refers to a microbiologic phenomenon where, if most members of a community have immunity to a contagious disease, the disease will be unable to spread. But if few members of that same community have innate resistance, then the disease will be free to run rampant—potentially with devastating consequences [50].

The vehicle of Boston's latest and most virulent outbreak came in the shape of a British Frigate, the "*Seahorse.*" In the autumn of 1720, His Majesty's Ship *Seahorse* weighed anchor from England and headed to the new world. Commanded by the ambitious 36-year-old Thomas Durrell, newly promoted to the *Seahorse*, the final destination was Boston. Newly built and commissioned that same year, *Seahorse* was a "sixth rate ship," of the Royal Navy [50]. The new frigate had a single deck with 20 guns, each capable of firing a six-pound cannonball. She was crewed by approximately 120 men, many of whom were conscripts and eager for a chance to jump ship at any opportunity.

Navigating in the southern channel past Little Brewster Island, the ship rounded the southern tip of Long Island, making its final approach to Long Wharf. To the starboard side, the ship passed Spectacle Island, two rounded hills connected by a thin spit of land in the shape of a figure-of-eight, looking from the deck as a pair of spectacles. Spectacle Island had been designated as the last stop for any fever ship approaching Boston. A primitive quarantine hospital, the Pest House had been built by order of the Massachusetts Assembly in 1717. Designated as a quarantine island for passengers with infectious diseases, the island was one method Boston used to minimize the spread of diseases like the Black Death.

The quarantine, however, was only loosely policed, since the last great plague in Boston had been almost 20 years earlier, from 1702 to 1703. The water bailiff's main rule was screening incoming vessels for contraband, and to ensure no foreign vessels entered the harbor, colonial trade being strictly limited to British vessels through the Navigation Act. Any merchant ship with a fevered sailor aboard was, in theory, required to hoist the red maritime "Q" flag, "quarantine" designating it as carrying pestilence, drop anchor off Spectacle Island, disembark the afflicted crew member to the Pest House and there await either their recovery or death. A further factor weighing against effective quarantine of incoming ships to Boston was the cost in further delaying arrival to the Boston warehouses, which lay tantalizingly close and within eyesight.

Ordered to escort a fleet of merchantmen to Barbados, the *Seahorse* took on board more than sugar, pineapple, bananas, and papaya during her four-week stay. As the crew mingled in the smallpox-ravaged island, a number became infected with the pox virus. Given an incubation period of about two weeks, it is likely many crew members were already dead before the *Seahorse* set sail back to Boston, probably dying on the island. Further, during the three-week return voyage, it is equally likely that the contagion flourished amongst the crew. Given the close quarters of the *Seahorse*, the contagion was certain to spread. Not surprisingly, during the stay in Barbados, the *Seahorse's* crew either went missing or died from mysterious circumstances, including desertion, but also smallpox. Upon arrival, the crew roster was examined by Boston authorities. Unsurprisingly, several crew members were found missing without a trace, obviously buried at sea. By the time the *Seahorse* had arrived in Boston on April 20, 1721, the ship had lost between ten and 20 sailors, certainly due to smallpox contracted in Barbados. And likely buried at sea to avoid scrutiny.

The *Seahorse* and Captain Durrell transported his contagion into
Boston where she anchored offshore from Long Wharf on April
20, awaiting a berth. The Boston water bailiffs were charged with
screening arriving ships for contagion, including Black Death and
smallpox, in order to protect the town from contamination. Captain
Durrell fully understood this. Despite knowing that many crew members
had died of smallpox, he selfishly anchored on Long Wharf to
gather provisions and necessary repairs from the Caribbean storm.
A law-abiding and compliant captain, of which Captain Durrell was
neither, would have been required to anchor at Spectacle Island.
Here, the sick would be transferred to the Pest House to avoid transmitting
the disease back into Boston. In quarantine, the ship would
lay idly at anchor. Rather than hoisting the red "Q" flag and transferring
any infected, Captain Durrell headed to port. Anchoring just
offshore, away from the prying authorities, several of the *Seahorse*
crew rowed ashore to visit the taverns and brothels of the town,
effectively guaranteeing the spread of the contagion into Boston [50].

Meanwhile, the disease took hold in Boston. The houses
stricken by the disease were kept in quarantine with makeshift
red flags posted at the door and put under 24-hour guard by the
authorities. The selectmen convened an emergency meeting and
ordered a door-to-door search of Boston to identify and quarantine
any further cases of the pox. From May 15 to 22, the search
found eight further eight cases of the pox. Worse, the cases were
scattered throughout the town, meaning the contagion was well
underway and almost impossible to isolate. On May 24, they sent
26 free Negros to decontaminate the streets with seawater, as a
preventive measure to contain the epidemic. By the middle of
June, the epidemic had a firm grip on Boston. The contagion so
gripped Boston that quarantining the sick was no longer possible,
and the speckled monster took hold[50].

About 1000 of Boston's elite fled the city in the hopes of avoiding the pox. William Tumane wrote to a friend in London, "The smallpox broke in and upon the City of Boston where it very much appeared with the terrors of death to the inhabitants."

Boylston

The Boston Puritan minister, Cotton Mather, was eager to rescue his reputation after his disastrous involvement in the Salem Witch Trials. An academic, prolific author, and son of the President of Harvard University, Mather was aware of Timoni's 1714 publication in *Philosophical Transactions*. His own slave Onelius bore a deep scar on his forearm from his inoculation as a child back in Africa. After Onelius had been exposed to the virus multiple times without developing the disease, Mather realized the inoculation did in fact work. Determined to salvage his reputation, Mather set out to introduce the practice to Boston. He first approached the only medically trained physician in Boston, Dr. William Douglass. A graduate of Edinburgh, Douglas dismissed Mather, preferring to rely on the contemporary treatments such as bloodletting and purging, the mainstay of smallpox treatment. There were several other self-proclaimed physicians, none of whom had any formal training, but had undergone some form of apprenticeship. Among these was Zabdiel Boylston, an ambitious 30-year-old self-appointed physician, who had apprenticed with his father Thomas Boylston, a local English surgeon. Zabdiel had first made his mark in Boston by performing the first mastectomy on a citizen with breast cancer and removing an enormous bladder stone in a 13-year-old boy. Turned down by Dr. Douglass, Cotton Mather approached the ambitious Boylston. Zabdiel did not think twice about the offer, and immediately started to implement the Levitan technique. A bonus to sweeten the deal was the fact that Boylston had already had smallpox, and was partially, if not completely, immune to the disease. He also had a personal agenda. As a small child, his family had been struck by smallpox, and Zabdiel had been sent out of Boston to live with a distant cousin. Several members of his family succumbed to the pox, leaving the young Zabdiel with a vendetta against the pox.

Boylston set to work implementing Cotton Mather's immunization treatment, starting with his 13-year-old son and two slaves. His son developed nearly-fully-fledged smallpox and narrowly escaped with his life. Following the Levitan technique, he made a small incision in the forearm and placed in pus from a victim of smallpox. Lacking walnut shells, Zabdiel used a warm cabbage leaf to maintain the inoculum in place, wrapping the site to seal the contaminant in place. The immunization produced a curtailed and weakened form of natural smallpox, lasting one to two weeks. Typically, ten to 20 pustules developed, compared to hundreds in the natural form, but these were shallower and more dried up earlier, producing no permanent scarring. The inoculation still produced fevers, body aches, and lassitude, but by no means as severe as the deadly natural smallpox.

In 1722, the epidemic was still raging across the city[50] So Boylston and Mather quickly reported the results of their campaign to a skeptical public. Of the 287 people inoculated by Boylston, only six patients, or 2% had died. Mortality in the general population was much higher: 844 out of 5,980 died (a 14.8% death rate). Publishing his results with his usual zeal, Mather showed Boston that the once risky practice actually dramatically lowered mortality rates. In 1724, Boylston traveled to London to present his results. Greeted by an enthusiastic scientific community, he went to the Royal Society two years later. Boylston Street in Boston remains a lasting legacy to the ambitious young Zabdiel. Boylston returned to Boston and died at the remarkable age of 89, rare in 18th century America. The probable cause of death was tuberculosis.

Jenner and the Milkmaid

In England of 1757, an eight-year-old orphan of a Gloucester vicar underwent the procedure himself. The young Edward Jenner would be responsible almost single-handedly for the mass immunization against smallpox using a more refined method, rather than the "hit or miss'" technique he had undergone as a child. Edward Jenner, born May 17, 1749, in Berkley, Gloucestershire, was orphaned at the age of five when his father, the Reverend Steven Jenner, passed away from tuberculosis. Brought up by his older brother, also a vicar, Edward attended school and was apprenticed to a local country surgeon in Sodbury near Bristol. At the age of 21, he became an apprentice to the world-famous John Hunter, one of the most famous surgeons in the land.

Based at St. George's Hospital in London, Jenner brought with him an unusual gift: many years of experience living with the local farmers in rural Sodbury. Because of this, he saw firsthand the ways of the local peasants and yeomen. It was well-known locally that the local milkmaids, exposed to the cowpox virus daily, never contracted smallpox. Thus, they somehow avoided the mutilated pockmarked face. Based on this information, Jenner figured the milkmaids had some innate immunity against the smallpox virus and set to work demonstrating this in the London population.

The story goes that in 1796, Jenner took cowpox tissue from the contaminated hands of a young milkmaid, Sarah Nelmes, and injected the contaminate underneath eight-year-old James Phipps's skin in an attempt to reproduce this innate immunity. This step was the world's first true vaccination other than the traditional smallpox inoculation. The child developed inflammation at the injection site, chills, and fevers, but recovered over the course of the next two weeks. Two months later, in July 1796, Jenner took an unprecedented and unthinkable step and inoculated the boy with fresh contaminates from a pustule on a smallpox victim. Instead of dying, as expected, the boy developed no symptoms. No swelling at the injection site, no reaction whatsoever. This convinced Jenner unequivocally that the child was now immune from smallpox.

Jenner named his new procedure "vaccination," after the Latin word for cow, the source of the cowpox disease. The following year, Jenner published his findings to the Royal Society of London; however, his publication received little interest in the medical communities. But Jenner persisted. Slowly but surely, the new method gained interest and was widely practiced more and more amongst the English physicians. As usual, professional jealousies arose in the shape of Drs. George Pearson and William Woodville, who worked at the local St Pancras smallpox hospital. Dr. Woodville, desperate to take credit for Jenner's success, found his own supply of cowpox pus from a sickened cow belonging to Thomas Tanner at the nearby Grays Inn Farm.

Woodville set to work, vaccinating 500 patients at his St Pancras Hospital, only to find almost all broke out in widespread pocks covering their bodies, rather than a single blemish at the injection site, which Jenner described from his vaccinations. Woodville's inoculum had obviously been contaminated with live smallpox virus, sickening hundreds and killing several. Jenner swung into action to defend his method and to discredit Woodville as a conniving blunderer.

Despite isolated campaigns to discredit Jenner, the effectiveness of vaccination continued to grow. By 1800, the technique was widely recognized as an effective way to combat one of the biggest killers in 18th century England. In 1802, in recognition for his work, Parliament awarded Edward Jenner £10,000, followed by £20,000 five years later. Vaccination proved to have two main benefits. First, using the less virulent cowpox virus had much more consistent results, and second, it resulted in much fewer deaths than the hit-or-miss transmission of live, virulent smallpox.

By 1840, the practice of variolation was made illegal. Known as the "father of vaccination," Jenner's life was not without its own tragedy. In 1810, his oldest son Edward died of tuberculosis, followed in short order by his two sisters, Mary and Anne, within two years of each other. A few years later, his wife also died of tuberculosis. Jenner died on January 23, 1823. His grave and his family's graves all lie near the altar of Berkley Church from whence he started.

Although the milkmaid's story is the standard and most imaginative explanation, an alternative explanation was related by Dr. Arthur Boylston in a 2018 edition of the *New England Journal of Medicine*: "The Myth of the Milkmaid."

Doctor Fewster and Farmer Jesty

According to Dr. Boylston, retired UK Pathologist, and no known relation to Boston's Boylston, in 1768, three decades before Jenner's experiment, a Dr. John Fewster was busy inoculating people with smallpox virus in a large house designed for that purpose, where they would stay until the typically mild cases of the disease passed. Part of his busy practice was a group of farmers in Thornbury, not far from where the young Jenner was an apprentice. To Fewster's surprise, some of the farmers whom he deliberately exposed to smallpox were already immune to the disease. There was no inflammation at the injection site, no chills, fevers, body ache, vomiting. The farmers reacted as if they had already suffered from smallpox and were immune. All denied any previous illness from smallpox. Absent also were the telltale pocks on the face, arms, and trunk, a sure sign of previous exposure.

Then, according to a letter Fewster wrote, one farmer said, "I have had the cowpox lately to a violent degree, if that's any odds." Fewster found that all the farmers who were not responding to the smallpox inoculation had never had smallpox, but all, to a man, had previously been infected with cowpox. He concluded that they were all immune to smallpox from exposure to cowpox. Fewster reported his discovery to the local medical society at their periodic meetings at the Ship Inn in Thornbury. Boylston's research was methodical and detailed. Examining documents dating back to the 1720s, he discovered the minutes of the Ship Inn meetings. In the list of attendees were two fellow practitioners, the Ludlow brothers. Although the 13-year-old Edward Jenner was not at the meeting, he was apprenticed to the Ludlow brothers in 1768.

Almost certainly, the inquisitive young Jenner must have heard accounts first hand from the Ludlow brothers during the course of his apprenticeship. He eventually became a member of the same medical society meeting at the Ship Inn. Subsequent minutes from the society's meeting over the years make reference to "the cowpox bore," Edward Jenner, for his obsession with Fewster's cowpox experiment. It would be 30 years before Jenner finally plucked up the courage to inject cowpox into the forearm of young James Phipps in 1796. The milkmaid explanation, although probably real, was likely Jenner's cover story for him to take all the credit for vaccination.

Another overlooked account of vaccination using cowpox, took place 20 years before Jenner's account. This pioneer was not even a physician, but a yeoman farmer, one Benjamin Jesty. In

1774, a smallpox epidemic encroached upon Yetminster, North Devon, home to Benjamin Jesty's modest farm. Over the years, Jesty was convinced that milkmaids who contracted cowpox from constantly milking cows became protected against smallpox. With an impending smallpox epidemic looming, Jesty took pus from the udders of his cowpox-infected cow's udders and transferred the material into the arms of his wife and two boys in an attempt to avert an imminent smallpox death. The attempt was successful, and all three survived. Not only that, but the process also conferred lifelong immunity from further epidemics of smallpox.

News of the controversial experiment percolated through rural England and eventually reached the skeptical ears of the medical profession, who decided on a bizarre and unbelievable confirmation of the technique. In 1805, Jesty received an invitation to visit the Original Vaccine Pock Institution in London. Accompanied by his eldest son Robert, already vaccinated 30 years earlier with the cowpox virus, he headed to the capital. The physicians, surgeons, and apothecaries of the Institution quizzed Jesty about his vaccination technique and, incredibly, insisted that Robert be reinfected with live smallpox to confirm the claims of immunity.

Robert accepted the challenge and was publicly re-inoculated with live smallpox virus to prove he was still immune from the deadly pox. Robert had no reaction whatsoever to the potentially deadly smallpox. No inflammation at the injection site, no chills, no fevers, no nothing. Conceding to Jesty's technique, all 12 of the Institute's examining officers were signatories to a statement of the "antivariolus efficacy" of his vaccinations. The statement was issued on Sept 6, 1805, and published in the *Edinburgh Medical and Surgical Journal*.

A portrait of Jesty was commissioned by the famous artist Michael Sharp. Disappearing in 1888, the portrait was tracked to South Africa, before being repatriated to London in 2005. A portulent Jesty smiles confidently from the three-quarter-length canvas, "a good specimen of the fine old English yeoman, dressed in knee breeches, extensive double-breasted waistcoat, and no small amount of broadcloth." The portrait now hangs in the Wellcome Collection of the Wellcome Trust in London.

PART THREE: BREAKTHROUGH

CHAPTER 8

LUCKY BREAKS

O n October 23, 1894, a farmer in the Oldenburg region of Germany returned home from the market with a newly pur-chased Friesian cow to add to his burgeoning dairy herd. Located in fertile grasslands in northwest Germany, Oldenburg was home to many of Germany's largest dairy farms. The black-and-white Friesian cow was native to the region, named after its pre-Roman region of Fresia. Sturdy reliable, producing large amounts of high-fat milk, and a proven reproductive animal, the Friesian was the work-cow, *"die milchkuh"* of the local dairy farmers.

Before long, it was obvious that the cow wasn't healthy. She gradually lost weight, developed copious liquid diarrhea, and her milk production dwindled. The farmer summoned local vet Herr Frederick Harmes to examine the cow. He saw the ravaged con-dition of the animal—her wasted ribs, prominent pelvic bones, ulcerated hide, sagging head, bony limbs, and bloated belly. The veterinary surgeon immediately suspected intestinal tuberculo-sis. Being aware of Koch's new skin test, the veterinary surgeon returned with tuberculin preparation and injected the cow's flank. To his surprise, returning a few days later, the cow did not show the florid reaction of inflammation, swelling, and sloughing of skin at the injection site, which was the diagnostic hallmark of tuberculosis. Neither did it show any signs of a cure, which at the time the tuberculin skin test was claimed to produce. The cow further deteriorated. As she slowly died, her liquid stool sprayed on the dairy pastures, and she progressively lost weight. Unable to stand, she gradually succumbed to pneumonia, slipping into debility. The cow died a wasting death weeks later, in the spring of 1895.

Herr Harmes was so puzzled by this odd case that he performed an autopsy on the dead cow and found the typical changes of intestinal tuberculosis, such as the inflamed and strictured intestinal mucosa, narrowing of the small bowel, and abnormal connections between adjacent loops of bowel. But missing were the huge, engorged lymph nodes in the mesentery of the bowel, the hallmark of tuberculosis. The cow certainly died a wasting death, typical of tuberculosis, but the ever-reliable tuberculin skin test was negative, and there were no fleshy lymph nodes in the cow's intestine. These findings didn't add up. What was this "new" disease? Herr Harmes sent specimens of the intestine to the veterinary pathology unit in Dresden, some 50 miles away. The cow's tissues were examined by Dr. Heinrich Johne and a visiting pathologist, Dr. Frothingham, from Boston. Under the microscope, the pathologists saw the typical changes of thickened mucosa often seen in tuberculosis. The intestinal wall was heavily infiltrated with white cells and giant cells and an unusual collection of white cells, a granuloma. Using an acid-fast stain, multiple red staining bacteria were seen infiltrating throughout the bowel wall in much the same way as seen in tuberculosis.

In an attempt to confirm that this new disease was TB, Dr. Johne injected tissue extracts from the bowel into guinea pigs, mice, and rabbits, repeating Koch's standard protocols used for over a decade to diagnose TB. He expected the animals to contract and die of tuberculosis, but they all thrived and failed to show any sign of the disease. The scientists were baffled. Dr. Johne concluded that although the culprit in the case was not tuberculosis, it may be a close species. Johne coined a new name for this new puzzling disease, *"pseudotuberculosis enteritis."* As in everything in medical science, the longer the name, the less is known about the disorder.

A campaign was launched to identify this new perpetrator, using extracts of dozens of known TB strains from scores of animals throughout the world, including mammalian, reptile, and avian. In 1906, a decade after Johne's discovery, a Danish veterinarian, Bernhard Bang, continued to work on the cause of this strange new disease. Although the infected animals failed to react to tuberculin antigens, and it was therefore not the classic TB, the animals did react to similar preparations prepared from the bird-sourced (avian) antigens. Bang proposed the disease be called "pseudotuberculosis," i.e., resembling tuberculosis, and coined the name *"enteritis chronic bovis pseudotuberculosis."* The names were getting longer. The problem was resolved later that year with a simple solution. The new disease would be named *"Johne's disease."* A new skin test was developed to test cattle, named *"Johnin test,"* since the equivalent test for tuberculosis was called "tuberculin test."

In 1879, with the advent of the new mechanical, suction milking machine for cows, replacing the age-old hand milking of cows, America imported a huge number of high-milk-producing dairy cows from Europe. The more efficient milking system was key to expanding a burgeoning dairy industry to serve a rapidly growing population. Highly productive dairy cows, Holsteins, Guernsey's, Jerseys, Ayrshires, and Brown Swiss cows, were imported en masse from Europe to America to feed the new industry. Unknown to anyone, also imported were cows with latent Johne's disease

A decade later, publications about the new disease, pseudotuberculosis enteritis or Johne's disease, soon appeared in the United States. The first case in America was described by Leonard Pearson in 1908. His paper "A Note on the Occurrence in America on Chronic Bacterial Dysentery of Cattle," published in the *American Veterinary Review* in 1908 detailed several cases in Pennsylvania, noting the similarity between intestinal tuberculosis. The cardinal difference between bovine intestinal tuberculosis and the new cattle disease was the absence of the typical caseous necrosis or cheese-like decomposition in the lymph nodes. Present, however, were the swarms of blue acid-fast bacilli, now easily recognized thanks to Koch's work. Frustratingly, and in spite of fastidious and persistent attempts at culture, the new bacterium refused to grow. What was this new mycobacterium? It certainly wasn't TB, because it could not be transmitted in the proven method of transmitting to guinea pigs or rabbits. It didn't produce the typical caseous necrosis in lymph nodes.

A New Killer is Identified: MAP

Having isolated, stained, and now even named this new superbug, the next hurdle was to culture it, to learn its strengths, and, more important, its weaknesses. In spite of repeated attempts to culture this organism, the efforts yielded negative results. Even the pickiest of eaters like Mycobacterium tuberculosis could be cultured in Koch's specific mediums if strict culture and temperature protocols were observed. But not even Koch's specific mediums worked on MAP. This new organism refused to grow. Period.

A lucky break came in 1912 when the British scientist F.W. Twort [49] continued to culture the new pathogen, again with repeated frustrated attempts. Twort, like many of his colleagues, was more scientist than a housekeeper. His lab was full of old petri dishes, contaminated flasks, and bacteria and specimen-strewn worktops. In the summer of 1912, Twort, glancing at a petri dish containing this new, unknown perpetrator, noted small bacterial colonies growing like satellites around the petri dish. Recognizing this as a new finding, Twort isolated the bacteria and was the first to report the successful culture of this new, acid-fast bacteria. This unusual finding was reported in the scientific literature, but nobody understood why it happened or what caused it. It would be decades later until Twort's good fortune was explained.

Twort[49] named his new bacteria, *"mycobacterium enteritis chronicae pseudotuberculosis bovis Johne."* As usual, the longer the name, the shorter the explanation. Twort went on to isolate other tissue from sickening cattle in England, and again reproduced the culture of his "new" bacterium. The culprit of Johne's disease had now been identified and could finally be cultured. Over the years, the bacterium was renamed "Johne's bacillus" and, in the 1990s, was finally christened *"Mycobacterium avium paratuberculosis"* or "MAP," back to its avian roots.

Decades later, Twort's puzzling success in culturing MAP was explained. Once more, it was due to a fortunate accident, and yet again, it was the result of an over-focused scientist failing to "wash his dishes." It was found that Twort's (unwashed) petri dishes had been left open to the elements and had been contaminated with a common hay bacillus "mycobacterium phlei" (Latin for grass), blown in through an open window from nearby hayfields. This mycobacterium phlei produces microscopic iron compounds known as siderophores. A nutrient secreted by certain bacterium, siderophores allow the entry of iron ions into the cell walls to enable their growth. Absent of this nutrient named mycobactin, the new bacillus was unable to grow. In the presence of mycobactin from the contaminated hay bacteria, the new bacteria started to grow and flourish.

The year after Twort's discovery of the MAP bacterium, in 1913, a Glasgow surgeon, Johnathan Dalziel[51], reported several cases of intestinal disease in his patients, which like the bovine disease, resembled intestinal tuberculosis. Dalziel's patients were thin, wasted, had abdominal cramps, bloating, diarrhea, and frequently died from an obvious intestinal malady. Autopsies of these afflicted patients revealed bowel inflammation, strictures, fistulas, and the cobblestone mucosa. Like intestinal tuberculosis, these lesions occurred throughout the GI tract, often skipping from one area to the next, so-called "skip lesions." However, absent was the caseous necrosis of tuberculosis, and the swarms of TB bacteria were nowhere to be seen. Noting the incredible similarity between this new disorder and the new pseudotuberculosis recently described in cattle (Johne's disease), he concluded: "the diseases may be the same." However, the absence of the acid-fast bacteria, found in swarms in the new Johne's disease, was puzzling. This was not TB for a series of reasons. One: because there were no bacteria. Two: there was no caseous necrosis. And three: the bacteria causing Johne's disease were nowhere to be found. Dalziel realized this was a new, devastating disease and called his new affliction *"hyperplastic tuberculosis."*

In 1932, the landmark article published in the *Journal of the American Medical Association* (JAMA) on October 15, titled "Regional Enteritis," [52] was published by three Mount Sinai Hospital doctors—Burrill Bernard Crohn, a 48-year-old seasoned gastroenterologist, Leon Ginzburg, a 34-year-old junior surgeon, and Gordon Oppenheimer, a 32-year-old budding urologist. Occasionally referred to as "the gang of three," sparks would fly over who performed the original research and who should be credited with the discovery. The 1932 *JAMA* article[52] described 14 more near-identical cases to those reported by Dalziel almost 20 years earlier[51].

The official position was that nobody was aware of Dalziel's publication. If this was correct, nobody had done their homework. Ironically, each case was provided by Mount Sinai surgeon Dr. A.A. Berg, who had operated on all of them. Berg declined, for reasons unknown, to have his name added to the list of authors on what was to become a milestone scientific article. The reasons would soon become clear as Crohn, Ginzberg, and Oppenheimer fought over bragging rights to the disease.

There were striking similarities between Crohn's 14 patients and Dalziel's three patients: there were no caseous lymph nodes that are so characteristic of intestinal TB, and there were no swarms of bacteria, characteristic of Johne's disease. This seemed to be a "third" disease, not intestinal tuberculosis, and not identical to Johne's disease. Nearly identical to intestinal tuberculosis, this "third" disease caused significant inflammation of the gut, fistulas, fissures, and a cobblestone appearance. However, missing were the swarms of acid-fast bacteria and the caseous necrosis found in every tuberculosis case to date. This disease looked more like Johne's disease. But where were the floods of bacteria? What was this new disease? Naming their new discovery *"regional ileitis,"* the first description of what would come to be known as Crohn's disease, hit the presses. The absence of any identifiable bacteria, as seen in intestinal tuberculosis and Johne's disease, would prove contentious for almost 100 years. In fact, it is still hotly debated today.

The absence of MAP bacteria in the tissue of Crohn's disease patients was a sticking point for decades. This central fact was always cited by the MAP skeptics. How could MAP cause Crohn's disease, if it wasn't even there? It would be another 50 years before a familiar name in the MAP debate revealed the answer. In 1986, Rodrick Chiodini published a bombshell article in the *Journal of Clinical Microbiology* titled "Spheroplast Phase of Mycobacteria Isolated from Patients with Crohn's Disease." The veteran researcher had examined cultures of Crohn's disease tissues which had been incubating for two and a half years. Even though there was still no sign of MAP's waxy coats with the conventional stains, Chiodini[18] discovered a cell wall-deficient form of the bacteria by the presence of its DNA. MAP had shed its thick, waxy coat to become a spheroplast or "uncoated" version of the bacteria. Finally, some answers to this conundrum. Here lay the answer to the absence of stainable MAP in Crohn's tissue. The bacteria were there, but they had removed their coats to avoid recognition. To remain viable, the MAP spheroplast hid inside the cells of the victim's tissue, an intracellular version of the bacterium. Not only was MAP safe from recognition using stains and culture, but it was also protected from the victim's own immune system, hidden within the cell itself. It was further discovered that even if MAP kept its coat, it could change from the typical "acid-fast" version to a non-acid fast form, essentially changing its color to avoid detection.

The eponymous naming of "regional enteritis" as "Crohn's disease" was not without its own drama. Ginzburg was quick to decry Crohn's involvement in describing the new disease with the accusation, "He (Crohn) played no role whatsoever in the development of either the concept, the research, the interpretation, or the writing of the original draft of "regional enteritis." Leading up to the drama, Ginzburg was a resident in Dr. Berg's surgical practice and had a particular interest in *"inflammatory granulomatous disease."* Because of this, he quickly accumulated 52 cases of the disease. He named his new disease *"segmental hypertrophic ulcerative stenosis of the terminal ileum."* Here we go again! Ginzburg recruited Oppenheimer, two years his junior, who at the time was an intern in the pathology department at Mount Sinai, to help him study this new disease and write a groundbreaking research paper. Somehow, possibly at Dr. Berg's suggestion, Ginzberg and Oppenheimer's manuscript was shared with Burrill Crohn (Figure 10), fourteen years Ginzberg's senior and certainly more politically adept than the junior, inexperienced underlings. Of the 14 patients with "regional enteritis," Ginzburg and Oppenheimer contributed 12 cases of the new disease, Crohn had two. Unannounced to all, Crohn presented the paper at the April 1932 American Medical Association meeting in New Orleans, omitting both Ginzburg and Oppenheimer's names. Outraged, Ginzburg approached Mount Sinai to correct this perceived intellectual theft. The committee, headed by Dr. Berg, resolved that the junior authors be added to the upcoming *JAMA* article[53]. But the damage was done. No records exist about the meeting, but apparently, it was also decided to list the authors by alphabetical order, luckily for Crohn. The following year, Ginzburg and Oppenheimer published their original 52 cases in *Annals of Surgery*[53], but Crohn's name was nowhere to be seen. There was certainly no love lost amongst the Mount Sinai "gang of three."

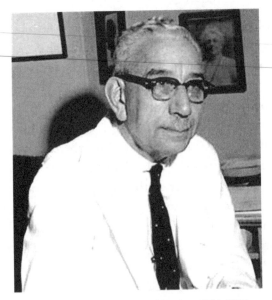

Figure 10. Dr Burrill Bernard Crohn. (1894-1993).

Burrill Crohn had a different take on the controversy, claiming that he and Berg had described all the cases, independent of his junior underlings. According to Walter Waggoner, who wrote Burrill Crohn's *New York Times* obituary on July 30, 1983, Crohn related the moment he was awarded the eponymous title of the "new" disease. At a GI conference in Prague, at least according to Crohn, a motion was proposed to call "regional enteritis" after himself. Apparently, Crohn rose to his feet to object to the motion, but he was ruled out of order and the name "Crohn's disease" was passed by unanimous acclamation.

Ironically, had Dr. Berg chosen to be involved in the controversy, and if the list of authors had still been listed in alphabetical order, Crohn's disease would now be known as "Berg's disease." Clearly, Dr. Berg did not need the drama.

IS900: MAP's Genetic Fingerprint is Discovered

Mycobacterium avium paratuberculosis (MAP) is notoriously difficult to culture, given its demanding culture requirements and temperature ranges, as well as a very slow doubling time, which is in excess of 24 hours compared to 20–30 minutes for the more common streptococcus or staphylococcus. This led to multiple erroneously negative results regarding the presence of MAP in biopsies of Crohn's disease. But, two factors improved the situation later. One: the development of PCR in 1984. Two: the description of a specific gene (IS900), which was specific for Mycobacterium Avium Paratuberculosis[27,54].

The technique of PCR involves duplicating the target gene, in this case in MAP, and amplifying these genes hundreds of thousands of times, where it can be detectable using electrophoresis. The DNA double helix for MAP, similarly in man, is a long chain of nucleotide bases (molecules), of which there are four. These are adenine (A), cytosine (C), guanine (G), and tyrosine (T). The DNA chain is made up of sequences of these nucleotides in a manner that is unique to each protein that is encoded by the unique DNA sequence. Imagine the DNA strand as a long string of beads with four separate colors distributed in a very specific and constant manner, so encoding for the specific gene product and producing a specific protein.

The DNA molecule is held together in a double helix by weak hydrogen bonds. The string of beads is distributed nose to tail, and each opposing base pair is held together by hydrogen bonds. The specific gene has a unique sequence, allowing us to identify it. In this case, Mycobacterium avium paratuberculosis was identified.

Human Genome Project

The Human Genome Project (HGP) was a 13-year, $3.1 billion project initiated in 1990 to sequence the entire human genome. Funded by the US Department of Energy and National Institutes of Health, and with collaboration from Britain, France Germany, and Japan, the project aimed to shed light on human evolution, identify the rogue genes responsible for hereditary diseases, and develop genome-based molecular medications against diseases such as cancer, diabetes, and, yes, Crohn's disease.

The human genome has 23 pairs of chromosomes, or 46 individual chromosomes, stored in pairs in the cell nucleus. The entire human genome is 3.2 billion base pairs long, or 6.4 million single bases, or individual nucleotides. There are approximately 20–25,000 genes in the human genome, each gene coding for a specific product or process. A small amount of total DNA, 1.5–2%, encodes for identifiable proteins, the building blocks of any organism. Let's refer to these as "product" genes. The remainder is often referred to as "junk DNA," equally certainly incorrect, as nature does not waste, replicate unnecessarily, or overproduce. Likely this DNA encodes for processes within the cell. Let's refer to these as "process" genes. For example, the sequence of gene expression, the rate of production, the "spell-check" genes (otherwise known as mismatch repair genes, when A and T mismatch, and C and G mismatch). These mismatch repair genes are very important in certain colorectal cancers, when the "spell check" mechanism breaks down, and pairing errors accumulate, resulting in faulty expression of the gene, and causes familial cancer, or Lynch syndrome. The MMR genes are tested in colon cancer patients, and are invaluable in identifying family cancer syndromes, identifying at-risk family members, and directing surgical and chemotherapy treatment modalities.

By comparison to the 26 pairs of chromosomes and 3.2 billion base pairs of the human genome, the yeast (Saccharides or brewer's yeast) has 16 individual chromosomes, consisting of 3.5 million base pairs, or seven million individual bases. This encodes and estimates 5,300 genes, compared to the human 20–25,000 genes. The yeast is a multicellular organism and contains a nucleus, which makes it a eukaryotic organism, like mammals, and even humans. Surprisingly, the yeast organism shares over 30% of its genomes with humans, that is over 30% of the yeast genome is identical to those found in humans.

Bacteria, on the other hand, are eukaryotic, single-celled organisms, whose genetic material is stored in a single circular chromosome, floating around in the cell's interior (cytoplasm) and lacking a defined nucleus. One of the most common and most studied bacteria, E. coli (sequenced in 1997) has 4.6 million base pairs, roughly nine million individual bases. and encodes for an estimated 3,000 genes

The MAP bacterium, a single-cell organism with a circular nucleus is like E. Coli, a prokaryotic, and shares many genetic similarities. Sequenced in 2006, the MAP bacterium possesses 4,829,781 base pairs, or almost ten million individual bases, and encodes for an estimated 4,350 genes. MAP shares 3,000 of its genes with its great grandfather, Mycobacterium tuberculosis. Within the MAP genome, the IS900 insertion sequence, made up of 1,451 base pairs, is critical in identifying the MAP organism much more reliably and with much greater sensitivity than the traditional culture or staining techniques[55]. The IS900 K10 sequence repeats itself in 15–20 locations within the MAP genome, thereby further amplifying the detection rate for the gene sequence and increasing the sensitivity of detecting IS900 in a PCR analysis, and detecting the presence of MAP in potentially infected cattle, environmental sources, milk and milk products, and even in tissue and blood samples of patients with Crohn's disease.

A string of base pairs, numbering over 1,400 in the insertion sequence known as IS900[27], has been identified and validated as specific for MAP. Fortunately, there are six or seven regions within the very long MAP genome in which the IS900 is repeated. The PCR process starts by unraveling the two chains of DNA by heating the DNA specimen to break the hydrogen bonds and separate the two DNA strands. This process of denaturing separates the two strands into separate, individual lengths of DNA. The process, a base pair, which is known to lie in direct proximity to the gene (known as the primer) is then added to the denatured DNA strands and attaches to the specific site adjoining the IS900 sequence, and attaches in a very specific, predictable, and reliable manner. After the cooling process to allow the primer to fix, known as annealing, the temperature is then raised. A new individual basis C, T, A, and G are added to the mix. The DNA sequence IS900 is then replicated by an enzyme, which creates an identical version of the gene, attached to a single strand. This polymerase enzyme is able to withstand heat in order to keep the DNA strands separate and therefore allow the replication, or extending process, to proceed. This enzyme, the Taq polymerase enzyme, is found in submarine thermal vents and is uniquely resistant to high temperatures and speeds the process of PCR. The three stages are repeated multiple times (20–40 times) and the specific gene or insertion sequence, therefore, is multiplied exponentially with each cycle. At the end of the PCR process, the insertion sequence can be easily identified by electrophoresis. The process of PCR and evolution in the identification of MAP is not only to avoid the unreliable process of culturing, which often takes several months, but to increase the reliability of identification of the MAP organism, and to enable this to be used in a field setting, such as testing for Johne's disease in an attempt to control the spread of MAP in dairy herds. IS900, the insertion sequence for MAP, is found to be reliable for several subspecies of MAP present in various animals, not only dairy cattle, but sheep, deer, and other agriculture animals. More importantly, IS900 has been identified in almost 90% of biopsies from Crohn's disease in intestinal biopsies[4,19], surgical specimens, and involved tissue. The identification of IS900 in Crohn's disease tissues led to a rethinking of the involvement of MAP in the causation of Crohn's disease[56].

Suddenly everything made sense. MAP had been in Crohn's tissues all along. It was not seen by conventional staining because these relied on the bacterium's waxy wall. Having shed its waxy coat, and entering the victim's own cells, using them as a refuge, it was invisible to the stains and microscopes of half a century of frustrated researchers. Inside the cell, MAP could wage mayhem on the victim's tissues for decades, never completely eradicated and free to emerge at any time to create another flare of the disease. If shed back into the environment, MAP was capable of restoring its coat back yet again. Alternatively, it could hide in other cells, such as the cells present in cow's milk, a major source of transmission of Johne's and Crohn's disease.

The fact that MAP could hide within white cells (inflammatory cells) in cow's milk had implications on the testing and pasteurizing of cow's milk. White cells are normally present in cow's milk, and since MAP was hidden within these cells, they could never be found by traditional staining and culture methods. This accounted for the negative results in isolating MAP in milk. Furthermore, the real incidence of MAP spheroplasts was almost certainly much higher than had been reported. Protected inside the milk's white cells also conferred a degree of protection against pasteurization, explaining the repeated frustration in completely eradicating the bacterium from the milk supply.

Not only was the prima donna bacterium a master of disguise, but it could also perform a disappearing act by shedding its coat altogether and hiding in its victim's cells. On top of this disappearing act, the bacterium could conceal itself within the "pus cells" of its victim's milk and escape its victim's dying embrace.

CHAPTER 9

CLUSTERS AND HOTSPOTS

There are many examples throughout the world where MAP-infected Johne's disease cattle are introduced into the indigent livestock, and after a latency of several years, the incidence of Crohn's disease spikes. These examples include diverse communities throughout the world, such as Winnipeg in Canada[7], Australia [8], Iceland [9], the Czech Republic [10], France [11] Minnesota [12], to name just a few. These diverse communities, many on opposite sides of the planet, have three underlying factors in common: MAP was introduced in some way, Johne's disease becomes endemic, and the incidence of Crohn's disease spikes, especially in locations where the disease was extremely rare.

In all of these examples, there is one repeating theme: MAP, then Crohn's. After Johne's disease and MAP have been introduced to herds of cattle, MAP proliferates in the exposed cattle and wildlife, such as deer[13]. Then, after approximately a 50-year latency period, Crohn's disease erupts. After this roughly five-decade latency, the incidence of Crohn's disease usually spikes to 25 times its prior rate and typically at an equally predictable rate of a fivefold increase in every decade. After 50 years, the incidence has reached a 25-fold increase, with no end in sight. Rather, the evidence points to a continued dramatic escalation of the disease.

As fast as Crohn's and Johne's disease are multiplying, research breakthroughs into the MAP-related diseases occur agonizingly slowly, not even close to catching up, or overtaking, the disease. It was in 1879 that Koch first obtained the tuberculosis bacterium [42]. It was almost a quarter-century later, in 1894, that Johne described the disease in cattle. Another 20 years would pass until Dalziel[51] described the first patient with what is today recognized as Crohn's disease, and a further ten years before Oppenheimer and Crohn[52] in 1932 let the general medical community accept Crohn's disease as a separate clinical entity. Almost 100 years later, we are still debating the cause of Crohn's disease[5].

The incidence of Crohn's disease is dramatically increasing in many parts of the world. In the Czech Republic, the incidence has increased five-fold since 1990, after they gained independence from the Soviet Union[57]. This is likely due to a change in international trade policies. As a result of the Czech Republic gaining their independence, there were unrestricted imports of subclinical cases of Johne's disease from the West into the newly liberated Czech Republic. Following the trend, Johne's disease flourished in the area for a few decades, long enough for the density of MAP to become well-established. Predictably, the incidence of Crohn's since 1990 has increased five-fold per decade[10].

In the southern hemisphere, Crohn's disease had been rare; hardly any cases were reported in clinical reports or epidemiologic data. After the introduction of MAP and Johne's disease, the incidence of Crohn's disease predictably spiked. After starlings were introduced to New Zealand and Australia[8], there was a predictable spike in the number of Johne's cases. Likewise, following this spike, the number of Crohn's cases increased in lockstep to almost 20 per 100,000, a predictable five-fold increase in the incidence of Crohn's disease[60].

In 1933, Iceland copied Scotland's age-old industry and introduced sheep as an economic stimulus to make better use of its vast, unused moorland. Thousands of sheep were imported, unfortunately carrying Johne's disease with them. Over the next few decades, Johne's disease and MAP were gradually transmitted to the indigent cattle herds, which leached into the retail milk supply and were consumed by unsuspecting Icelanders. From 1933 to the 1990s, the incidence of Crohn's disease has spiked by an alarming 18-fold increase[9].

Not only is the incidence of Crohn's disease increasing, but there are several known pockets of the disease, "hotspots," of dense concentrations of Crohn's scattered around the world on at least four continents. In these same hotspots, the incidence of Johne's disease has spiked to levels never previously seen. Interestingly enough, in these same locations, MAP has been isolated in much denser concentrations in the environment: the water supply[56] (such as lakes and reservoirs) and the food chain (like dairy products and indigent dairy herds).

The Contaminated Rivers

In Cardiff, South Wales, Crohn's disease has had the same explosive growth[58,59,61]. The incidence in Cardiff is likely due to contamination of Johne's infected cattle from the Brecon Beacons, a high-density agricultural region around Cardiff. Contaminated effluent is washed by the heavy Atlantic storms into the local river, the Taff, which flows through the center of Cardiff. The incidence of Crohn's disease in the last several decades has shown the customary five-fold increase from 50 years ago[58]. Surprisingly, the densest concentration of Crohn's disease is in 11 wards (districts), eight of which border the river[59]. The remaining three lay leeward to the Taff. When samples were taken from the river and surface foam, they were cultured for MAP. The data from the PCR results demonstrated a high incidence of MAP in both the river water and surface film, leading to the conclusion that MAP was aerosolized and blown by the prevailing southwestern winds. Not only that, it was also blown to the shorelines and leeward (northeastern direction). More worrisome, water samples from local reservoirs and even domestic drinking water were also positive for MAP.

In Minnesota, the incidence of Crohn's disease is stable at about eight per 100,000 inhabitants. Four hundred miles north, the incidence in Winnipeg[7] is nearly four times that: 30 per 100,000. The reason? The Red River flows north from Minnesota into Winnipeg and supplies a significant amount of the drinking water. When tested for MAP, the Red River showed positive. As in the Cardiff scenario, this is likely a result of contamination from the grasslands in the Midwest of the USA, which drain into the Red River and flow north into Winnipeg. More alarmingly, these clusters also focus not only on an individual city, but on the same street. In one example, two families along the same street in Winnipeg had a mother, wife, and two siblings affected by Crohn's disease in an alarmingly short three-to-five-year interval. A neighbor several houses down the street has no less than seven of their 11 children affected by Crohn's disease. There was no previous family history of the disease. Not surprisingly, MAP was isolated in the drinking water supplying the entire street.

Along with the steady rise in Crohn's in many parts of the world, there are also several reported hotspots of the disease, where dense concentrations of the disease are reported out of the blue, with no prior history of the disease. In 1993, a report[11] appeared in the journal *Gastroenterology*, titled "A Study of Crohn's Disease in Two French Families." The report detailed two families in northwest France, one living in a small town, the other a small villa 12 miles away, in which 12 children developed Crohn's disease. There was no prior history of the disease in either family. In the first family, the father developed Crohn's disease in 1970, followed four years later by two of their four children, each within several months of each other. In 1982 and 1983, the other two children developed Crohn's disease followed by their mother, five years later. In the second family, seven of the 11 children developed Crohn's disease, four of the children within ten months of each other, then six years later another child, then six years later, two more siblings. In 1970, there was no PCR available, so IS900 assays were not performed. At the time, MAP was suspected, possibly from a local milk source, but was never confirmed.

In 1992 in the village of Bleckley, a rural community of about 2,000 people in Gloucestershire, England, 12 people developed Crohn's disease between 1960 and 1983, a 6.7-fold increase. The village, which had its own water supply from local springs, lay in a hollow surrounded by upland pastures grazed by cattle in which clinical Johne's disease was evident.

In New Zealand, Crohn's disease has risen dramatically, from a rare disease to one of the highest in the world. A "cluster" of the disease is found in the Canterbury region of South Island with Christchurch as its principal city[21]. Mountains are to the northwest and rivers from them run across rich agricultural pastures and either side of Christchurch before entering the sea. A small river meanders through the city itself and was identified as the likely source of MAP contamination.

A further cluster occurred in the town of Mankato, Minnesota[12], USA, and involved the occurrence of seven cases of

Crohn's disease amongst 285 graduates of the Mankato West High School class of 1980. All seven had been swimming in local ponds, lakes, and the Minnesota River, just downstream from the Blue Earth River estuary, whose catchment included rich agricultural grazing land. Evidence points to the likely heavy contamination of these waters with MAP.

A further example of the transmissibility of Crohn's disease is demonstrated in the migration of individuals from a low-incidence Crohn's disease population into a higher, usually urban environment with a high incidence of Crohn's disease. These low-risk, non-contaminated, uninfected individuals adopt the high rate of Crohn's disease in their new native environment. With the dramatic increase in the incidence of Crohn's disease in such places as Cardiff[58,59], the Czech Republic[57], Stockholm[62], and Christchurch[60,69,79], New Zealand argues definitively against a primary genetic role for Crohn's disease and a clear role of MAP in propagating the disease.

Milk is collected and stored in bulk before packaging and distribution as consumer milk products in urban areas. Only a few contaminated cattle may therefore contaminate a very large amount of bulk milk, leading to potential transmission to thousands of individual consumer products. Likely for this reason, the incidence of Crohn's disease is dramatically greater in urban areas compared to rural populations. Control of MAP in milk products is obviously important in controlling spread to the consumer. More important is the control and elimination of MAP and Johne's in domestic dairy cattle herds. The incidence of MAP-positive herds in North America is reported as high as 70%–90%.[63,68] The incidence of MAP in milk in spite of pasteurization has also been reported as high as 3%–5%[14,64-66]. In much the same way as bulk storage of milk increases the risk of transmission of MAP in the retail milk supply, management of infected Johne's disease stool, which is bulk stored as slurry, may also increase and multiply the incidence of MAP contamination in the environment.

Liquid slurry is spread by agricultural tankers on to the grasslands as a source of fertilizer. Therefore, only a handful of infected cows in a herd of possibly hundreds can distribute MAP through the grasslands. Moreover, effluent from the contaminated grass flowing into the River Taff in Cardiff, into the Red River in Winnipeg, and many other rivers throughout the world can introduce MAP to human water infrastructure. Once MAP spreads to these rivers, it leaches into reservoirs and eventually domestic tap water. Just as MAP is not susceptible to standard pasteurization of milk, MAP also resists usual chlorination procedures used to decontaminate reservoir supplies, resulting in MAP turning up in tap water sources in cities such as Cardiff [59], Winnipeg[7], and Christchurch, New Zealand[21,60].

The Rats of the Sky

The European starling (starling vulgaris) is a medium-sized black bird with a glossy black coat and a wingspan of about eight inches. The starling is one of the prime suspects as a vector of MAP and the global propagation of Johne's and Crohn's disease [24,80]. Blackening the sky as they fly, the bird is endemic to Eurasia and flies in flocks of millions of birds. The birds migrate from central Eurasia in the fall to the cooler climates of Scandinavia and northwestern Europe. A map of their migration overlaps exactly the highest distribution of Crohn's disease in the northern hemisphere[33]. Estimated at hundreds of millions, the starling population continues to multiply in spite of attempts to cull and eradicate the species.

Overflying the grasslands on their path of migration, massive swarms of starlings drop cumulatively hundreds of tons of contaminated droppings on the pastures of Norway, Sweden, Denmark, Britain, France, and Germany. When this happens, the grazing pastures are thoroughly contaminated. As the domestic dairy cattle graze on the grass, they consume the contaminated grasses and become infected. The starling is a scavenger. Dense flocks are a common sight in the feeding troughs of the local domestic cattle and sheep in the grasslands of northern Europe. Depositing the contaminated feces containing MAP into the feeding troughs of the dairy herds is a near-certain mechanism for transmitting MAP into the dairy and subsequent milk supply.

A 2005 study from Minnesota, published in the *Journal of Dairy Science*, titled "Applied and Environmental Microbiology" by Joseph L. Corn[66], examined 30 species of free-ranging birds and mammals on livestock premises in the State of Minnesota. Thirty species of wild animals were examined, including the rat, the deer population, possum, raccoon, skunk, and shrew together with the European starling. Not surprisingly, the starling was found to have one of the highest prevalence of MAP in its gut compared to three other avian species examined.

Further studies in 2016 and 2014 examined the distribution of MAP in Minnesota and Canadian dairy farms. The studies[63,68], published in the *Journal of Dairy Science* reported positive cultures for MAP in 80% of North American dairy farms, in locations from cow alleyways, manure storage sites, carving areas, cow pens, liquid manure spreaders, and water runoff. The highest incidence was reported in the densest concentration of the cows and in the manure slurry pens, which pool liquid stool from hundreds of cows.

The starling has few natural predators. The much rarer hawks, owls, and harriers do little to cull or even stabilize the hundreds of millions of starlings flying around Scandinavia and northern

Europe[80]. A map of the migration patterns of the starling looks like a copy and paste version of the map of Johne's disease and Crohn's disease[24]. Unfortunately, in the 1800s, the starling was also exported to the United States, Australia, New Zealand, and South Africa. In 1890, Eugene Schieffelin imported 60 common starlings to New York City and released them in Central Park. Schieffelin was president of the American Acclimatization Society, whose goal was to introduce every bird species mentioned in William Shakespeare's works into North America. Lacking predators and thriving in a dense urban environment like New York City, the original 60 birds swelled to hundreds of millions across North America and Central America.

Similarly, a misguided campaign was devised by Cecil Rhodes, who imported the common starling into South Africa in 1897. Rhodes's motive was to introduce the starling as a measure against insects plaguing the burgeoning South African agricultural economy. Again, lacking few natural predators, and protected as a misguided measure against crop insects, the starling population exploded in South Africa. Likewise, Johne's disease and Crohn's disease followed in lockstep, neither of which had hitherto been experienced.

In 1857, the starling was introduced to Australia for the same reason—to guard against insects. Australian farmers also wanted to pollinate their crops in their burgeoning agricultural economy. Nest boxes were built. Food abounded. Few predators existed. It's no wonder that the population quickly exploded. By the turn of the century, the starling was a common sight in Victoria, Queensland, and New South Wales. Realizing the mistake, people quickly relabeled the starlings as pests, the rats of the sky. As the incidence of the starling population burgeoned, so, predictably, did the incidence of Johne's and soon, predictably, the incidence of Crohn's disease started creeping up from a rare disease to one of the most common GI complaints in Australia and New Zealand[60,69].

A few years later, the starling was introduced into New Zealand to control the caterpillar pest consuming their crops. In 1862, the Nelson Acclimatization Society nurtured the bird, which rapidly morphed from protector to pest. New Zealand, has one of the most rapidly increasing incidences of Crohn's disease, especially in children, with the likely culprit from MAP droppings from the starling into the dense dairy herds of New Zealand, and then finding its way into the milk supply and environmental sources such as rivers, lakes, reservoirs, and tap water[67]. The map of the migration path of the common starling as well as its newfound homes in the U.S., South America, Australia, and New Zealand is stark and disturbing evidence for the role of Johne's disease, MAP, and ultimately the starling vulgaris as the perpetrators for Crohn's disease.

CHAPTER 10

GOT MILK?

In the late 19th and early 20th century, bovine TB was endemic in the cow herds of Europe, and the bacterium was transmitted in cow's milk. The TB-infected milk was consumed by millions of European children, entering their intestines and resulting in intestinal tuberculosis. This resulted in the narrowing of the bowel, perforation into adjacent organs, rupture of the intestines, and if you were lucky, a quick and agonizing death from intestinal perforation. The unlucky victims were doomed to a slow and agonizing death from gradual starvation, abdominal pains, intractable vomiting, impossible cramping before bowel perforation, and death, as happened in 65,000 children in England and Wales between 1912 and 1932.

TB attacked other vital tissues; it could also contaminate the glands of the throat, causing "scrofula." Scrofula is a massive enlargement of the neck glands, which often erodes into neighboring arteries after a victim vomits their entire bloodstream in a rapid exsanguinating death. Often, the glands ruptured through the skin of the neck, resulting in a hideously deforming and scarring of the neck, not to mention draining pus constantly. Additionally, the glands would often rupture into the trachea (windpipe), dripping a constant flow of pus into the lung. If the victim did not die from the paroxysm of coughing, pulmonary (lung) TB would ensue, thereby sealing the victim's fate.

If the glands perforated into the esophagus (gullet), the victim would choke, vomit, and gag on their own spit. Usually, this resulted in a slow starvation death, where the victim was unable to swallow and aspirated fluids into the lungs, ending in a long, consumptive demise. Any of these scenarios could and would transmit the TB to the lungs, resulting in constant coughing, hacking, choking, inability to breath, wasting, fevers, and a slow, lingering death. If the disease eroded into the major vessels of the chest (aorta or inferior vena cava [IVC]), the victim would drown on their own circulating blood, a mercifully quick but horrific end.

TB was controlled in Europe by a combination of herd culling and milk pasteurization. The introduction of pasteurization was effective in destroying bovine tuberculosis, hence making the milk supply safe and slashing dramatically the incidence of tuberculosis and deaths in children. Between this and an aggressive culling program of affected farm animals, TB was eradicated in milk and was probably the major factor in ridding Europe of TB. Currently, the incidence of infantile or childhood intestinal tuberculosis from milk is almost never seen, a direct consequence of the success of the cattle TB screening, culling, and pasteurization programs.

Pasteurization
Following Koch and Pasteur's work on sterilizing tuberculosis, pasteurization became widespread in the UK in 1922 as a result of the Milk and Dairy Act, which required pasteurization of all milk. Similar measures were enacted in the US. First in 1947 and then later in 1973, when the US federal government required

pasteurization of milk shipped across any state line. The combination of screening herds for tuberculosis, culling of infected tuberculosis cows, and widespread milk pasteurization has resulted in a dramatic decrease in bovine tuberculosis. A vaccine or drug therapy is only for the few who have fallen through the gaps in the process. A similar protocol must be enacted to eradicate MAP from the food supply, starting with widespread cattle screening, culling infected animals, and screening of milk for the MAP bacterium. In the unlikely advent of a vaccine, it will likely be too little too late. Even the introduction of RedHill Pharmaceutical's RHB-104 will be not a preventive measure but used only to treat those who have fallen through the gap and succumbed to Crohn's disease.

Pasteurization of milk may take various forms and with variations in temperatures and duration of heating. The original technique was 50 degrees Celsius (100 degrees Fahrenheit) for five minutes. This proved completely inadequate, and MAP was soon found to be more heat resistant as a result of its thick, waxy coat. Therefore, pasteurization to kill MAP was increased to 62 degrees Celsius (144 degrees Fahrenheit) for 30 minutes, so-called VAT pasteurization, for large quantities of milk.

With the introduction of the high temperature and short-time pasteurization (HTST) method, the most common method used, the temperature was increased to 72 degrees Celsius (162 degrees Fahrenheit), but only for 15 seconds. This was still nowhere near adequate to kill mycobacterium paratuberculosis[70-72]. Paratuberculosis can survive 15 seconds at 90 degrees Celsius (194 degrees Fahrenheit). By living within the cell, and protected by its thick, waxy coat, the MAP was able to survive temperatures hitherto not considered for pasteurization.

In 1993, veteran MAP hunter, Professor Herman Taylor, and Dr. Rodrick Chiodini identified living MAP in pasteurized milk, even milk pasteurized by HTST[72]. The finding placed the pair in the lime-light, if not the crosshairs, of the Ministry of Agriculture Fisheries and Food (MAFF) in the UK[20] and the US Department of Agriculture (USDA) in the US. In 1996, the finding was independently confirmed in Australia. Two years later, it was confirmed in the US[31]. Quickly becoming a political and public issue in Europe and the US, the effectiveness of pasteurization in killing MAP was a hot topic[14].

In 1993, it was time for some damage control. First, the CA Milk Processor Board hired the San Francisco advertising company Goodby Silverstein and Partners to launch a campaign to boost milk consumption. The resulting campaign, "Got Milk?" was an icon of the advertising industry, which ran for over 20 years. In 1995, the campaign went national and was licensed to the National Milk Processor Education Program (Milk PEP). During its 20-year run, "Got Milk?" featured over 350 celebrities: entertainment icons like Whoopi Goldberg, Taylor Swift, Naomi Campbell, sports celebrities like Serena and Venus Williams, Reggie Bush, and even imaginary celebrities such as Kermit the Frog and the Simpsons. A "Got Milk?" Barbie Doll was even launched by Mattel. The celebrities, models, actors, actresses, and athletes alike were shown drinking a glass of milk with a "milk mustache." Although immensely popular, the campaign met with limited results. Consumption of liquid milk actually dropped from 0.96 glasses per day in 1970 to 0.59 glasses in 2011, a result of the increasing array of sodas, fruit drinks, energy drinks, and bottled water. People for the Ethical Treatment of Animals (PETA) countered the campaign with their own: "Got Pus? Milk Does."

Public Panic

In light of recent events, the MAFF swung into action. In 1998, the European Union (EU) undertook a study to test samples of retail pasteurized milk off of a grocery shelf for living MAP[7]. Ireland was chosen because of its increasing incidence of Crohn's disease, its dense dairy farming industry, and its high milk consumption. Researchers went to 16 retail stores and purloined 31 cartons of milk from a variety of sources. The researchers were shocked when six of the 31 samples (19%), grew live MAP[7]. A public relations crisis and press uproar immediately followed. There was a national outcry in Ireland and Europe, which pitted the dairy industry, the Department of Health and Agriculture in Britain, and the public at large in a contaminated milk scare. The press reports immediately alerted the British people that drinking milk could cause Crohn's disease. The public panic was immediate. In response, three of the largest supermarket chains in Britain (Sainsbury's, Safeway, and Tesco) assured the people that the pasteurization protocol would be increased from 15 to 25 seconds, an increase of ten seconds. Unfortunately, none of this was based on any facts, and the new technique was soon found to be inadequate. Meanwhile, the British government swung into full defensive mode. The British minister of agriculture went on live national TV to drink a glass of milk in front of the cameras, and announced, "I drink pasteurized milk, and it is safe to do so with confidence."

Shortly after, the "Irish" experiment was repeated in Britain, when researchers went to a number of stores, taking hundreds of samples of retail pasteurized milk off the shelf.

Over a 17-month period (March 1999 to July 2000), a total of 814 cows' milk samples were tested: 244 bulk raw and 567 commercially pasteurized (228 whole, 179 semi-skim, and 160 skim), from 241 approved dairy processing establishments throughout the United Kingdom. Testing showed *Mycobacterium paratuberculosis* was present in the milk, identified by PCR in 7.8% of raw milk samples and, more worrisome, was found in 11.8% of pasteurized milk [64]. After several months of painstaking culture, live MAP was found in 1.8% of retail pasteurized milk. The results caused public panic, and was devastating news to the dairy industry.

Early in 2000, the US Animal Health Association met to discuss the spreading panics and what they should do about it. They decided that the USDA should replicate the Irish and British studies and test retail dairy products in the US. The National Milk Producers Federation member, John Adam, vocally opposed this measure, declaring, "The FDA has already stated their position, they are confident that the pasteurized milk is safe, and we do not need to test retail milk." But the Para-Tuberculosis Awareness and Research Association, http://www.crohns.org, another public advisory group, pushed back against this statement. Steve Merkel, a founding member of the organization, and whose wife suffered from Crohn's disease, retorted, "With all due respect sir, if milk is as safe as you stated, then retail testing will simply confirm the fact," and, "Are you afraid of retail milk testing because you are afraid of what you might find?" But the resolution on testing retail milk in the US was overwhelmingly rejected.

In 1998, the USDA acquiesced to public pressure and developed their own experiment[74]. The USDA pasteurized fresh milk at 15 seconds at 72 degrees Celsius; however, they first pretreated the milk to high-frequency sound waves as well as freezing. This way, they could weaken, if not kill, any contained MAP. The resulting milk was then pasteurized to the standard 72 degrees for 15 seconds, resulting in, not surprisingly, a negative result[73]. The head of the USDA, Joseph Smucker[75], went public to announce, "The results indicate the transmission of live paratuberculosis TB by pasteurized milk is unlikely. After a review of the available literature on the subject, it is the position of the FDA that the latest research shows conclusively that commercial pasteurization does indeed eliminate the hazard." The scientific community was quick to identify the flaws in the flawed experimental technique and a scientific uproar resulted in multiple letters to the editor [70,71,74]. This process was never performed during routine HTST pasteurization of milk, and the implications of a "rigged" experiment were obvious. The experiment didn't represent reality.

Shortly afterward, the University of Wisconsin, independent of the USDA, studied the presence of MAP in retail milk[65]. A total of 702 pints of retail whole milk were purchased in three of the top five milk-producing states (233 from California, 234 from Minnesota, and 235 from Wisconsin) over a 12-month period and were tested for the presence of viable MAP. The criteria used for identifying samples as positive for viable MAP were a positive PCR with a subsequent positive culture. The results revealed MAP in 11.8% of samples by PCR testing and viable MAP in 1.8% of the retail whole milk pints tested. Of the 22 brands of retail milk tested, 12 (55%) yielded at least one sample positive for viable MAP, so this was not a flawed pasteurization process: The problem was a resilient and resistant MAP, which was not entirely eliminated by pasteurization.

What the researchers were not expecting was the seasonal variability of MAP in milk, which directly mirrored the same seasonal variability of Johne's disease and also Crohn's disease. The number of samples containing viable MAP was similar among states, and there was a seasonal variation in the presence of viable MAP in retail milk. More MAP-positive samples were identified during the fall and winter months, compared to other seasons.

Just as MAP has a seasonal cycle, every disease has its own cycle. For example, influenza flares in the winter, typically in elderly individuals. Likewise, whooping cough (pertussis) flares in the fall and winter in infants. During the winter months (specifically

September through February), hospitals are inundated with influenza cases, and hospital beds are hard to come by. Because of this, elective surgeries are difficult to schedule. Similarly, pneumonia peaks during the winter months (specifically November through February) and has the same repercussions with overwhelmed hospital admissions. The seasonal change in the exacerbations of Crohn's disease is well known and was detailed in a 1996 paper by Zeng and Anderson on seasonal variation in inflammatory bowel disease. The authors studied 139 patients with Crohn's disease over a 20-year period. In a total of 10,693 follow-up months for these patients, 592 relapses occurred. The highest relapse rate was found in the autumn and winter, whereas the lowest was in the summer. The authors concluded that Crohn's disease has seasonal exacerbations with flare-ups in the fall and winter months. This is not to suggest that MAP was transmitted to de novo cases of Crohn's disease during those short few months. Rather, MAP has the same inherent cyclic seasonal rhythm as many other diseases do, like flu, pneumonia, croup, and whooping cough, to name a few. Whether manifested by Johne's or Crohn's disease, MAP behaves in the same way.

Eradication of MAP from the Environment

The eradication of MAP will need to follow the eradication of its progenitor, *mycotuberculosis bovi*. Prior to pasteurization, the tuberculosis was transmitted in milk and caused the death of some 65,000 people between 1912 and 1937 in England and Wales alone. The bovine tuberculosis, present in raw milk, is ingested by the victim. The bacterium then invades the intestinal wall, usually the terminal ileum and cecum, causing intestinal tuberculosis. Patients suffered the typical signs of obstruction, strictures, inflammation, perforation, and death. The control of bovine tuberculosis is not only at the origin itself, i.e., infected cows with tuberculosis, which involves screening of the cows, culling infected cows, and also milk pasteurization. Vaccination against tuberculosis was performed in England, the UK, and Europe, but with questionable protection. On the other hand, subsequent drug therapy is expensive, lengthy, and only used in those victims who have slipped the safety net and developed intestinal tuberculosis. The same strategy must be performed to eradicate MAP from the environment. The first step must be to educate patients with Crohn's disease and the medical profession about the role of MAP in Crohn's disease. They are, after all, the individuals suffering from this horrific disease, whilst their physicians, equally unaware, are left to battle its consequences. Second, there must be public awareness about the dietary and environmental sources of MAP, in a disease that affects 1.5 million Americans, many more millions worldwide. Precedents abound, such as the role of tobacco in causing lung cancer. Finally, and eventually, government agencies such as the CDC, USDA, European Union[33], and UK Department of Health[20] may accept that Crohn's disease is a zoonotic disease transmitted by MAP from birds to cows and finally to humans via contaminated milk and other environmental sources [5,36]. Any denial of this, and there will be no significant federal funding. This step is essential because this is the greatest source of research funding and eventual drug registration.

Next, screening programs of domestic dairy cows and milk for MAP must be routinely implemented and bolstered. Current screening programs have failed to decrease, far less eliminate, the problem. Early culling of infected animals and early weaning of calves could potentially diminish the source of MAP in the milk supply. Screening of milk is already practiced but clearly needs bolstering. Unfortunately, relying on a MAP vaccine to solve the problem is unlikely to be feasible any time soon. But the advent of a therapeutic drug in the form of RHB-104 is a glimmer of hope for those patients with Crohn's disease who have fallen through the cracks.

With the death of tens of thousands of children in England and Wales, a program of eradication of bovine TB was launched in the UK in October 1950. It consisted of tuberculin skin testing of dairy cattle and slaughter of cattle reacting positive to the skin test. While this has led to a dramatic decrease in bovine tuberculosis in England and Wales, the disease has shown a recent resurgence. This is possibly due to the infection of dairy cattle by badgers, whose population is increasing in England and Wales and are a known source of tuberculosis. As a result of this resurgence, about 40,000 dairy cattle were slaughtered in England and Wales in 2019 alone.

CHAPTER 11
THE MAP HUNTERS

I f we are to implicate MAP as the cause of Crohn's disease, we should at least turn back to Robert Koch and his four principles[55]. If you recall, these principles are used to establish that a specific disease is caused by a specific bacterium[18]. His first principle was that the bacterium should be present in the diseased animal or individual, but not in uninfected, healthy ones. Second, the bacterium should be able to be purely isolated and cultured. Third, transmitting the bacterium to a healthy, uninfected animal should cause the identical disease; and fourth, the bacterium should be able to be isolated in the newly infected animal. We will now look at each of these principles in relation to MAP causing Crohn's disease.

To reiterate, Koch's first principle states that the responsible bacterium should be present in abundance in affected individuals. Through spheroplasts, the MAP-Crohn's connection has been proven many times, meeting this first principle. This has been primarily proven through the use of the IS900 PCR test. Initially, skepticism against the MAP-Crohn's connection centered around the fact that the bacteria could not be seen using conventional

stains under light microscopy. This fact confounded investigators from the time of Dalziel and Crohn. How could MAP cause
Crohn's disease if it wasn't even there? This was a valid question.
Because of this seemingly inconclusive data, the theory that there
was a connection was dismissed, and continues to be dismissed to
this day. But we know now that the bacterium is exceedingly difficult to find in tissue samples since it has a thick, waxy coat which
is almost impenetrable to common bacterial stains. This has made
the identification of MAP in samples of intestines resected from
Crohn's disease patients extremely difficult.

In 1986, the veteran MAP hunter Rod Chiodini discovered
why MAP could not be found in Crohn's tissue using conventional
staining[18]. This is because MAP had a trick up its sleeve. When
it enters its human victim, it sheds its thick, waxy coat. The cell
wall deficient version, called a spheroplast[18], was basically just the
DNA. With the advent of PCR, the genetic fingerprint, IS900[26,27],
was found and was identified in practically every Crohn's disease
tissue examined, even in their blood. Like any *Cold Case* or *CSI* episode, MAP had been positively identified as the culprit. With this
data, it should have been a closed case. Unfortunately, the original
skepticism was hard to leave behind, and the dogma that MAP
cannot be seen, using a microscope, in Crohn's tissues persists to
this day.

The second of Koch's principles states that it should be possible to purely isolate and culture the bacterium. This has been
satisfied many times over, either as the 20th-century interpretation of isolate and culture or as the 21st-century interpretation of
Kohn's criteria, i.e., the PCR identification of IS900 oligonucle-
otide sequence. As we have seen, MAP, like its great grandfather,
mycobacterium tuberculosis, requires an extremely specific culture medium at a very specific temperature (38 degrees Celsius).

Even when these conditions are met, MAP's doubling time is over 24 hours, compared to 20 minutes for a common bacterium such as E. coli. Despite these difficulties, pure cultures of MAP can be obtained, albeit after years of incubation and using very stringent temperature and medium requirements. When we apply modern criteria for identifying MAP, i.e., IS900, the data that MAP is present in Crohn's tissues is widespread and undeniable

The third principle requires both transmission to a healthy animal and reproduction of the disease. In 1984, a research biologist at Montana State University, Rodrick J Chiodini, an outspoken and controversial pioneer in the MAP "conspiracy campaign," reported the first successful transmission of Crohn's disease to a second healthy animal. A key step in meeting Koch's third principle, Chiodini "fed" Crohn's infected intestinal biopsies to healthy infant goats[25]. A radical and controversial, but necessary step. The "oral inoculation," as it was euphemistically described, of the MAP-laden Cohn's tissue resulted in the goats developing intestinal Cohn's disease in approximately five to six months. The earliest lesions occurred in the ileum and consisted of granulomas in the intestinal walls, the diagnostic hallmark of Crohn's disease. The goats went on to develop all the classic features of human Crohn's disease.

To satisfy the final and fourth principle, the same bacterium must be reisolated from the experimental animal. Indeed, acid-fast bacilli were found in the intestines of the experimental goats and tested positive for MAP. All four principles had been proven. Case closed. Having satisfied Koch's principles, we also need to take it a step further. Not only should the microscopic evidence be considered, but the macroscopic, global epidemiologic evidence should also be evaluated[22-24,56].

To evaluate the global, epidemiologic evidence, there are four more principles to consider. These four principles are ones I created based on Koch's principles, our "macro-principles," reiterated in epidemiology or transmission evidence. First, the bacterium responsible for the disease and the disease itself must occur and be found in the same location worldwide. Second, an increase in the responsible bacterium should lead to a similar increase in the disease. The third is transmission. There must be a proven mode of transmission from the bacterium to the victim. Fourth, the bacterium should be isolated in the victim's tissue.

Macro-principle #1: Koch's four principles are echoed by demographic findings reflecting the close association between Johne's and Crohn's disease. Firstly, an increase in the prevalence of the reservoir of MAP, i.e., Johne's disease is a lockstep with an increase in the number of Crohn's disease sufferers[56]. It is known conclusively that Johne's disease is caused by MAP. The incidence of Johne's disease, according to the US Department of Agriculture, is increasing dramatically over the decades. According to a study in 2000, dairy herds were screened for the bacterium and showed the presence of MAP in 20–40% of herds screened. A more recent study in 2018 was performed and reported that 80–90% of herds contained at least one MAP positive (Johne's) cow. During the same period, the incidence of Crohn's disease has increased dramatically; in some locations, such as South Wales, it has quadrupled

This increase in the incidence of Johne's disease has stimulated the agricultural community, the USDA, and specifically the Johne's disease research bodies to call for more aggressive screening and culling of diseased cows.

Echoing Koch's third principle, we need a means of transmission from a diseased animal to a healthy animal, or individual. The mode of transmission from the bird vector to cattle is well known. The source of mycobacterium paratuberculosis is within migrating birds. After all, the word avium is Latin for "bird," and the disease is found most commonly in migrating birds. MAP has been routinely identified in the stool of the migrating flocks of birds, the most common perpetrator of which is the common starling. The starling may be the winged vector, but the vast "reservoir" of MAP resides in Johne's contaminated dairy herds.

Johne's and Crohn's Go Global

After its first description by Dalziel in 1912 and Crohn in 1932, the incidence of Crohn's disease was most prevalent in Scandinavian countries, Northern Europe, the US, and Canada[22-24]. The most plausible theory is migrating birds swarm across the Northern Hemisphere shedding their MAP-laden droppings on the grazing pastures of these countries. The Northern Hemisphere contains the highest incidence of grasslands, and therefore, the greatest density of grazing dairy cattle. These same areas coincide exactly with the highest density of Johne's disease in cattle and Crohn's disease in humans[56].

Along the equatorial regions of the globe (North Africa, Asia, and Central America), the arid climate does not support pasture lands and the hot, dry climate cannot sustain large densities of milk-producing cows. The equatorial regions are home to the driest parched areas of the globe, the Sahara Desert, the Gobi Desert, Accordingly, the incidence of Crohn's disease in the equatorial belt is much lower.

A further element of the Northern and Southern Hemisphere argument centers on the rising incidence of Johne's disease, and in turn, Crohn's disease in Australia, New Zealand, and South Africa. Fifty years ago, Crohn's disease was rare in these regions. There is now an alarming increase in Crohn's predominantly affecting children and adolescents[21-24,77,78]. This is the likely scenario[19,20].

At the beginning of the 20th century, the starling was introduced into Australia, New Zealand, and South Africa to control insects and caterpillars which were ravaging their crops[80]. Lacking any natural predator, the starling's population exploded, and so did the rate of their MAP droppings of the pasturelands below. The mode of transmission starts with the reservoir of MAP bacterium from massive flocks of migrating birds, primarily the starling, which drop their MAP-laden droppings on the grazing pasturelands. Then grazing dairy cattle ingest the MAP in the contaminated grasses, and the cattle develop Johne's disease[13,56].

After the once-healthy cows develop Johne's disease, they are wrought with profuse, watery diarrhea, which sprays over acres of pasture-like faucets. This in turn transmitted MAP to the rest of the grazing herd, in a continuous, repetitive, and never-ending cycle. Johne's is also transmitted from the diseased cows to their newborn calves through their udders, as the calves suckle their mother's milk. This in turn infects the newborn calf in an almost unstoppable cycle if the problem is not recognized. Unseen and imperceptibly, Johne's disease flourished in the cattle herds, transmitting their MAP into the retail dairy products, milk, cheese, and yoghurt consumed by the hitherto healthy children in Australia, New Zealand, and South Africa[56].

The transmission of MAP from newly introduced starlings to cattle is a series of progressions that typically takes several decades. First, the starling population has to explode to adequate numbers to sufficiently contaminate pasturelands. Then, a certain number of cattle have to be infected with Johne's disease. This entire process typically takes 50 years, which lines up with when starlings were introduced (1900) and when the number of Johne's disease cases spiked (1950). After Johne's disease is established, another few decades pass, about 50 years, until the spike in Crohn's disease is noticed, so around 2000. The scientific literature abounds with alarming reports of the escalating incidence of Crohn's disease around that time [22-24,56].

Once even a single cow has contracted Johne's disease, the resulting diarrhea sprays the MAP, with disproportionately greater effect and efficiency, over greater areas of grassland. This, therefore, acts as a second mechanism of multiplying the spread of MAP, thereby affecting a greater number of cattle in an ever-repeating, self-perpetuating cycle. As the cows rest on the grassland, the stool is frequently contaminated on the cow's udders which, if adequate cleansing methods are not undertaken prior to milking the cow, can lead to direct fecal to milk transmission of the bacteria, without even transitioning through the cow.

The presence of the (MAP) bacterium in the milk supply, therefore, has a plausible, but until recently, unproven track. In a 1997 USDA study of 2,500 dairy herds in North America, 20–40% of cows were found to be positive for MAP. By 2020, a similar study showed that 90% of US dairy herds contained at least one MAP positive (Johne's) animal. The increased intensity of the dairy industry means that there is more concentrated grazing of cattle herds on dairy pasture. This is one factor that has been put forth as responsible for the increasing incidence of Johne's disease. In an intense, high concentration of dairy farming, the milk from each cow is combined together, often from hundreds of cows. After the milk is combined, it is pooled in refrigerated vats, often containing thousands of gallons of milk. The bulk milk is stored and remains cooled for pickup by bulk milk tankers, commonly on a daily basis. As these bulk milk tankers travel from dairy farm to dairy farm, the milk from any single MAP-contaminated cow can contaminate many thousands of gallons of milk.

This bulk collection and storage from hundreds or potentially thousands of cows are then distributed as retail consumer milk, in gallon or quart cartons. The milk from any single MAP-contaminated Johne's cow may therefore end up in multiple batches of retail milk. It is therefore easy to see how a few contaminated cows may contaminate massive amounts of bulk stored milk, and after industrial processing and packaging, contaminate multiple cartons of retail milk.

The Rogue Genes

The argument does not obviously suggest that everyone who drinks milk will develop Crohn's disease. It is well known that Crohn's disease has a hereditary basis. The disease runs in families, and there is a high rate of the disease in identical twins. In 2001, two studies were published in *Nature*[82], identifying the gene NOD2 that causes some people to be predisposed to Crohn's disease[83]. Later, the NOD2 gene was renamed CARD15[84]. The studies revealed that the CARD15 gene was responsible for the defensive properties of the mucosa against MAP[83]. Within the CARD15 gene, there are two sites (domains) that defend the intestinal mucosa against MAP and other invading bacteria. The first domain, LRR ((leucine-rich-repeats), codes for a protein that recognizes invading pathogens, including MAP, and attaches to their outer coats. The second domain, CARD (capsane recruitment domain), enables the intestinal mast cells to kill the bacterium, essentially swallowing the bacterium (apoptosis). It is basically a one-two punch orchestrated by the CARD15 gene[85].

Two normal copies of the CARD15 genome (homozygous, or one on each of the two DNA strands) would therefore convey cellular immunity against MAP if it were ingested. Any anomaly in one (heterozygous) or both (homozygous) CARD15 genes, conversely, would be unable to prevent the entry of the MAP bacterium into the intestinal wall[86]. Entering the intestinal cell, it creates a florid immunological reaction, resulting in a cellular hallmark of Crohn's disease, the granuloma, as well as the clinical findings of strictures, fistulas, perforation, and cobblestone mucosa.

If only one CARD15 gene is defective (heterozygous) there is an approximately two-fold increase in Crohn's disease. If both CARD15 genes are defective (homozygous) there is an approximately 20-fold risk for the disease. Not only is there a far greater risk of developing Crohn's disease with a CARD15 defect, but the disease, if developed at an earlier age, was more aggressive, and typically developed as ileal disease[87], the most common form of Crohn's[88].

The MAP-Crohn's conspiracy, therefore, takes a further step, explaining the familial trend of Crohn's. If MAP is ingested through contaminated milk by a healthy, CARD intact individual, the innate intestinal immune systems deploy, and MAP is destroyed by LRR and CARD proteins. If the same contaminated milk is ingested by an individual with a defect in one or both CARD15 genes, the intestinal defense mechanisms are defective. Because of the hole in the intestinal defenses, MAP penetrates the intestinal defenses, causing the inflammatory mayhem of Crohn's disease, like strictures, fistulas, perforation, and cobblestone mucosa.

PART FOUR: A CURE FOR CROHN'S

CHAPTER 12

SMALLPOX REDUX: A CROHN'S VACCINE

MAP is purely an intracellular bacterium and cannot survive outside the cell in animals, humans, or milk. The vaccine, therefore, needs to enter the interior of the cell in order to generate an adequate type 1 immune response. The Jenner Institute at the University of Oxford has a long and successful track record using attenuated adenoviruses, the cause of the common cold. Unfortunately, MAP vaccinations to prevent Crohn's disease are in the very early stages and do not show a great deal of promise. The effort is being spearheaded by Professor Herman Taylor and his daughter, Amy, a primary care doctor. Since no federal government agency recognizes the causative relationship between MAP and Crohn's disease, it is not eligible for substantial federal funding. The USDA refuses to accept MAP transmission to humans as a cause of Crohn's disease and the CDC makes no mention of it on their website www.cdc.gov. Because these organizations refuse to accept this probable cause, funding for the vaccine primarily comes from private donors, patients with Crohn's disease, and friends and families of patients. A few concerned individuals periodically donate too. The Crohn's and Colitis Foundation of America, is a 50,000-member, highly organized, and motivated group of Crohn's sufferers, families, friends Physicians, and industry groups are reliable, but purely voluntary and altruistic sources of research funding. So, it's not enough.

The sparse funding, estimated at £850 thousand over the last ten years of their endeavor, a drop in the bucket compared to typical multi-million vaccine development, has also been supplemented by Dr. Amy Taylor, a self-confessed non-athlete, running marathons, and other fundraising measures. Professor Taylor's website advertising and promoting the MAP vaccine (www.HAV-vaccine.com) has a large prominent button titled "DONATE" in order to supplement what were essentially meager donations from the general public. Most importantly, if the federal government agencies refuse to accept Crohn's disease as transmitted from animals (a zoonotic disease), there will be no substantial federal funding any time in the near future.

Since humans frequently develop common colds from adenovirus, the original trials using human adenovirus vectors were unsuccessful, because the virus vector was recognized by the recipients' existing antibodies created from previous bouts of colds caused by human adenovirus. The virus vectors were therefore rapidly destroyed by the patient's immune system and were ineffective. Accordingly, a simian (chimpanzee) adenovirus was substituted, which was not recognized by the recipient's immune system and therefore survived to carry its payload inside the cells.

The adenovirus is a live, attenuated vaccine, similar to the development of the tuberculosis vaccine. This renders the virus incapable of reproducing within the human body, and potentially creating an adenovirus cascade spreading its lethal payload with disastrous results, similar to the tuberculosis vaccine fiasco which led to the Lübeck disaster. The attenuation of the virus results in the deletion of 20% of its genetic code, rendering it incapable of multiplying, i.e., non-replicating.

The viral vector is designated ChAdOx2 (acronym for Chimpanzee Adenovirus Oxford), the vaccine antigens. Added to the ChAdOx2 virus are key components of the MAP genome, two from the cell surface and two from cellular secretions to maintain the cell wall. Collectively these are referred to as the HAV antigens[89] and are present in all MAP bacteria, ensuring complete coverage of MAP bacteria and leaving no MAP bacteria undetected, therefore avoiding destruction. The ChAdOx2 then carries its HAV payload inside the macrophage to generate a T cell response against MAP.

After the initial vaccine injection ("the primer"), the recipient's first line of cellular immune defenses (the macrophages) identify the "foreign" adenovirus, and engulf the ChAdOx2 package, complete with the MAP HAV antigens. In the second phase of the immune response, the macrophages display the HAV antigens on their cell surface, to present the intruder to the circulating T cells and to generate a tsunami of T cells to kill any and all HAV antigens (and MAP) in the recipient's circulation. T cells are the key component in the immune system that attacks intracellular invaders, as opposed to the B cells, which produce circulating antibodies. Since MAP is a purely intracellular pathogen, a T cell response is required to destroy the MAP hiding within the victim's cells.

A second "booster" vaccination is given six-eight weeks after the initial ChAdOx2 primer. Since the recipient's immune system is now "sensitized" to ChAdOx2, a second injection with the same delivery system would be immediately destroyed, and therefore be ineffective. A second viral vector is therefore used for the booster dose, this time a weakened (attenuated) pox virus, Modified Vaccinia virus Ankara, "MVA"[90]. The MVA vector was initially developed in Ankara, Turkey, by culturing vaccinia (pox) viruses from inoculating the pox virus in goat and donkey skin, a throwback hundreds of years to Jesty, Fester, Jenner, and Boylston's smallpox vaccinations.

Through hundreds of "passages" through culture media, the virus becomes progressively weaker. The attenuation process results in attenuation by deleting 10% of MVA's genetic code, in order to prevent it from replicating[91]. This genetically modified virus is also incapable of multiplying within the recipient's system and, like ChdOx2, is a harmless, non-replicating indolent viral "mule" used to carry the HAV payload into the recipient's macrophages and generate a further tsunami of anti-HAV T cells to seek out and destroy any MAP hiding within the recipient's body. The Jenner Institute's adenovirus vector model has been successful in HIV and Ebola vaccines and is the same methodology used in the Oxford/AstraZeneca model for the current Covid-19 vaccine, which is now being used around the world.

The Jenner Institute at the University of Oxford and Professor Taylor have published three early trials related to the immune response of the vaccine and its safety. The first vaccine trial was performed in mice and showed some modest stimulation of the mice's immune system against MAP. A subsequent study in cattle showed a similar boost in the cattle's immune system, and decreased shedding of MAP in the cattle's stool, but was largely disappointing.

In a subsequent human study, three groups of volunteers were injected with three different doses of the vaccine. Disappointingly, of the six patients receiving the largest dose of vaccine, only two showed a significant increase in the immune response to MAP[92].

A second human trial in Crohn's disease patients was started in the fall of 2019, also run by the Jenner Institute, using the same virus methodology.

The goal of the latest trial in Crohn's disease patients is to decrease the severity of the disease. The outlook, because of scant funding, the disappointing results in mice, cattle, and early human trials, gives little reason for optimism in the vaccine trial against MAP. Adding to the gloom, the outbreak of the Covid-19 pandemic has put the trial on hold. The true goal of a vaccine that will prevent susceptible individuals from developing Crohn's disease is, optimistically, many years away.

Professor Hermon-Taylor summarized his frustration and anger against the establishment on "Crohn'sMAPvaccine.com." In a posting titled "Censored – The Crohn's connection," Hermon-Taylor put it succinctly: Now we've got a bug that you can't see, can't grow, hides under the immunological radar, is a bastard to kill, and the problem it's causing is far, far greater. If Rod Chiodini and I are wrong, the magnitude of the problem will only be the economic losses of farm animals, which is costing the U.S. somewhere between $1.5 and $2 billion a year. If Rod Chiodini and I are right, then, oh dear, oh dear. We have a big problem. It's going to take a lot to put it right.

CHAPTER 13

MAGIC BULLETS

Paul Ehrlich, a contemporary of Robert Koch, was present at Robert Koch's famous Friday evening presentation to the Physiology Society of Berlin on March 24, 1882. Ehrlich, nine years younger than Koch, went on to discover the first effective syphilis antibiotic, known as Salvarsan. The German Ehrlich joined the prolific German chemical conglomerate, Interessengemeinschaft Farbenindustrie AG, commonly known as IG Farben (dye industry conglomerate). The Germans, taking full advantage of their vast chemical industry infrastructure, were years ahead of their European and American competitors. Capitalizing to full advantage on imports of oil from their African colonies, the Germans dominated not only the petroleum industry, but also the resulting dye manufacture and ultimately a burgeoning and rapidly evolving antibiotic industry.

Following Koch's presentation, Ehrlich studied the selective uptake of dyes by bacterial cells compared to human tissue. Experimenting first with methylene blue, he noted the higher uptake of the dye in bacterial cells compared to the background uptake by the human tissue cells. A byproduct and widely recognized side effect of his experiments were his characteristic blue fingertips from handling the many samples of methylene blue.

His cardinal belief was that if the bacteria took up the toxic dye selectively, they may therefore succumb to these toxic chemicals and be used in what he called "chemotherapy" for bacterial infections. Ehrlich coined the term "magic bullet" to kill bacteria. His first successes came with treatments for treponema pallidum, causing syphilis; trichinosis, endemic in Africa and causing sleeping sickness; puerperal fever, causing thousands of postpartum deaths in German mothers; and, of course, the elusive tuberculosis.

Ehrlich tested thousands of byproducts of oil distillation and extraction in search of his magic bullet. Also investigating the compound arsenic, his chemists produced hundreds of compounds based on the arsenic compound. In 1909, he tested compound 606, arsphenamine, later to be called Salvarsan[93]. In his lab, he showed the compound was toxic to treponema pallidum, the cause of syphilis, then endemic in Germany and Europe.

Smallpox was differentiated from its sister plague "The Great Pox" or syphilis, then prevalent in Europe. Syphilis, a sexually transmitted disease, starts as a small, painless nodule, a chancre, on the penis, vagina, or around the mouth, and lasts a few weeks. Months later, the secondary stage emerges as a "copper" colored rash on the hands or feet. Years later, anywhere from two to 20 years, the tertiary stage evolves, as inflammatory nodes (gumma) develop in the brain, causing "insanity," on the shin bones, causing "bow legs," and often on the bridge of the nose, resulting in the telltale "saddle nose" deformity. Death inevitably followed as it did in the case of Lord Randolph Churchill, father of Sir Winston Churchill, at the age of 45.

In 1912, Ehrlich tested his new "chemotherapy" on 31 end-stage cases of syphilis, all demented from the disease. Miraculously, all reported dramatic success. Many even recovered their mental capacity. But his studies were interrupted by the outbreak of World War I in 1914, when imports of his antibiotic to Britain and eventually to the US were banned. After his experience with Salvarsan, it was obvious that the compound, which contained 32% arsenic, was toxic to its human recipients, causing multiple deaths[93]. Nonetheless, it would be the mainstay of treatment for syphilis throughout Europe until 1945, when penicillin became more widely available, providing a less toxic and more effective treatment for the disease.

In 1932, Gerhard Domagk, another German-trained chemist, tested an oil derivative with a characteristic red tinge, widely used as an azo dye in the German chemical industry. Testing the red dye on mice, he noticed that the mice suffering from streptococcus or staphylococcal infections responded to the red dye and survived. For first time in history, there was a potentially effective treatment. The new red dye, Prontosil, received a skeptical reception from the medical community until 1936 when the son of President Roosevelt developed tonsillitis and was expected to die. Desperate for any treatments to save his son, President Roosevelt insisted that his son receive treatment with Prontosil. The child survived, and Prontosil received a huge public relations and economic boost. The simple red dye would become the progenitor of a major class of antibiotics, the sulfonamides, still widely used today as Bactrim and Septra, to name but two.

Domagk spent much of his early career with IG Farben, the German pharmaceutical conglomerate, including the Bayer Company. The Bayer Company was already famous, and flush with cash from its production of aspirin, (aminosalicylic acid), derived from willow or poplar bark. This acid was one of the earliest analgesics and antipyretics (fever-lowering medications).

Domagk eventually became the director of Bayer with its blockbuster aspirin product; however, Prontosil was never a commercial success since its patent had expired prior to the discovery of its antibacterial properties.

Subsequent French researchers discovered the parent drug Prontosil was actually a "prodrug," and the active compound was a derivative, which they called sulfanilamide. Various derivatives of the new sulfanilamide were developed and are still in production and clinical use today. Currently, the one most commonly used today is cotrimoxazole (Bactrim) to treat urinary tract infections and HIV infections. Domagk was awarded the Nobel Prize for his discovery in 1939, but with Hitler and the Nazi Party in power, he was arrested by the Gestapo and instructed to refuse the prize, which was regarded as "un-German." Later, in 1947, after World War II was over, he was able to accept the Nobel Prize.

"Mold Juice"

In 1928, a little-known British chemist, Alexander Fleming, inadvertently discovered the penicillin class of antibiotics, in his now-famous petri dish culture of streptococcus and staphylococcus. As the story goes, Fleming left his petri dishes on the windowsill of his lab at St Mary's Hospital London, open to the elements, rather than placing it in an incubator, as was the standard practice. Leaving on a two-week vacation, Fleming returned to his lab and retrieved his neglected petri dishes. To his puzzlement, he found clear zones around deposits of yeast, which clearly had killed the streptococcus and staphylococcus colonies. The standard explanation was that Fleming had left the open petri dishes on his window ledge, where fungal spores had settled, leading to its discovery. In reality, it is highly unlikely that Fleming left on a two-week vacation leaving his windows open and the petri dishes uncovered, exposed to the London weather. The less romantic, but more likely, explanation is that the fungal spores drifted up the stairwell from the laboratory beneath Fleming, where experiments on fungi were being actively researched. He named his new antibiotic, Penicillin, after the strain of Fungus, Penicillium, which caused this seemingly quirky phenomenon. Although not recognized at the time, his discovery was one of, if not, the most important discoveries in the history of medicine, if not mankind.

But Fleming's discoveries went largely ignored at first. Although they were published in an obscure publication, the *British Journal of Experimental Pathology* in 1929[94], his article received little attention and was unnoticed for another ten years. In 1939, the Australian Howard Florey and Russian Ernst Chain discovered Fleming's publication and started to expand on discoveries. The bombastic Florey, whose father had emigrated to Australia from England to "cure" his wife and two daughters from tuberculosis, used his energy and ambition to work his way back to England. By 1938, he was head of the Dunn Laboratories at Oxford University, charged with developing penicillin for use in the looming World War II. In 1933, the equally volatile and temperamental Ernst Chain, a Russian-German Jew, fled Germany to England, leaving his family, who ultimately perished in the holocaust. Ending up at the Dunn Laboratories, the Florey and Chain partnership proved to be historic, though volatile.

At Oxford University, penicillin was produced by a process of fermentation, requiring the presence of oxygen. The mold therefore only grew on the surface of the fermentation "juice" and was collected by skimming the precious mold from the surface. This required massive areas of fermentation space, and every conceivable vessel was recruited into service, including bedpans. The campaign soon took over a large portion of the medieval university grounds. Eventually, by March of 1940, enough penicillin was produced to perform toxicity tests, to establish if the drug would be life-saving or lethal. Chain injected two mice with the new drug. Thankfully, both survived unharmed. Now onto more testing. Having passed its toxicity test, hemolytic streptococci (obtained from a new mother with puerperal fever) was injected into eight mice on May 25. Four of the mice were subsequently injected with penicillin. Sixteen-and-a-half hours later, the untreated mice were dead, and the four mice that had received penicillin were alive and well.

Early in his career, Florey received a Rhodes scholarship and spent time in the US, where he made valuable connections with the US medical community and USDA. Due to the USDA's massive fermentation resources, this connection would prove critical in the industrial fermentation of penicillin. Florey recruited the British drug giant ICI (Imperial Chemical Industries) to produce penicillin, but it soon became clear that many more resources would be required. So, Florey recruited US corporations into a consortium to enable penicillin to be fermented in industrial amounts. By the time the Pearl Harbor attack occurred in November 1942, Florey had assembled four major US drug companies to focus entirely on penicillin production: Merck, E.R. Squibb, Charles Pfizer, and Lederle Laboratories. Together with dozens of American universities, the USDA and Department of Energy (DOE) produced 2.3 million doses of penicillin available for D-Day in June 1944.

But the German-developed sulfasalazine also played a critical role in D-Day. Ironically, the antibiotic powder shown being sprinkled into soldiers' wounds in epic movies such as *Saving Private Ryan* was not the Allies' penicillin, but the German sulfa-based drug. On D-Day, each Allied soldier carried a small packet of powdered sulfasalazine in their rucksack to help sterilize penetrating gunshots, shell fragments, or knife wounds, so delaying the onset of overwhelming sepsis, and enabling the victim a few hours or days grace to be transported for surgery.

After the war, the ambitious Chain left Oxford and Florey to join the Institute Superiore di Sanita in Rome, where he continued to synthesize the penicillin molecule and adapt it to its second-generation molecules, ampicillin, and Penicillin-V. Subsequently, these would evolve into third and fourth-generation cephalosporins, all based on the original penicillin molecule. Given his German roots, Chain's emphasis lay in industrial manipulation of the molecule, rather than Florey's approach of fermentation. Returning to Imperial College, London, Chain's genius ultimately proved the more successful method and spawned the drug company, Beecham.

Later, it was excitedly discovered that penicillin could be used as a cure for gonorrhea, syphilis, puerperal fever, cellulitis, and many other common gram-positive bacterial diseases. But unfortunately, it was ineffective against any and all gram-negative infections, including cholera, typhoid, anthrax, and, of course, the elusive tuberculosis[95].

TB "Wonder Drug"

The breakthrough in the search for a tuberculosis antibiotic came in 1943 at Rutgers University. At that time, most major universities were seeking new and groundbreaking antibiotics from the same source as Fleming had done with penicillin, from Mother Nature herself. A leader in the search for natural antibiotics, Selman Waksman was a world expert in soil bacteria and fungi, principally the fungus Actinomyces. Interestingly enough, he was also a Russian-Jewish immigrant. Actinomyces was found in decomposing soil, manure, and compost, permeating its surroundings using fine hyphae while secreting one of the most primeval and potent natural antibiotics. Working from his Rutgers base, Waksman received assistance from Merck Laboratories, also in New Jersey, to produce an antibiotic with activity against human gram-negative organisms, as well as potential biological threats from the Nazis. Waksman had isolated the antibiotic streptothricin, which was active against typhoid, but when injected in experimental mice and guinea pigs, it killed the animals outright. This toxicity, therefore, excluded it as a potential antibiotic in humans.

In 1943, a 21-year-old graduate student, Albert Schatz, arrived on Rutgers campus as the understudy for the famous professor Waksman. Also the grandson of Russian-Jewish immigrants, Albert was a zealous, meticulous, and dedicated student who would ultimately be the principal investigator in the discovery of the new antibiotic streptomycin. Streptomycin was active not only against the gram-negative organisms, but also the elusive tuberculosis. In the end, for his discovery of streptomycin, Schatz was rewarded with ridicule from Waksman and a lawsuit from Rutgers University. In his book, *Experiment Eleven. Dark Secrets Behind the Discovery of a Wonder Drug,"*[92] Peter Pringle, a *New York Times* and *Washington Post* writer, describes the discovery of streptomycin, together with the resulting battle between Schatz and the combined forces of Waksman and Rutgers University.

Albert was assigned to work in the Department of Soil and Microbiology to analyze multiple sources of the actinomyces fungus, a potential antibiotic for tuberculosis. Because of the perceived dangers from the presence of live tuberculosis in his lab, he was strictly confined to the basement of Rutgers University. From a hive of experimentation on soil organisms, animal droppings, and compost, Schatz extracted samples from various sources of topsoil, compost, and manure. He even obtained samples from the throat of a chicken, donated by a colleague, Ms. Doris Jones. The basement was the hive of cultures from multiple sources and multiple subcultures from those sources. Proving to be a fairly constant presence within topsoil, animal droppings, and stable manure, actinomyces was a fruitful source of potential antibiotics for the ambitious Albert Schatz.

On the morning of August 23, 1943, Albert Schatz started his famous experiment 11. In a meticulous laboratory notebook, Schatz entered control soils #2, #17A, #18A, straw compost, leaf compost, and stable manure. All were plated out on egg albumin. At the end of his entry, he wrote, "some actinomyces obtained from the plates of swabs of chickens' throats, from Ms. Doris Jones." Albert labeled the two samples 18-16, which means the 18th subculture from sample 16, and D-1, the D for Doris, the source of the chickens from which the throat cultures were derived. By mid-September, two strains of actinomyces were growing, each of them a gray-green color, which he named Griseous, Latin for gray. Albert applied samples of 18-16, and D-1 Actinomyces to petri dishes containing typhoid and cholera germs. To Schatz's excitement, a clear patch appeared around the samples of 18-16 and D-1, indicating that these new antibiotics were killing typhoid and cholera, producing clear "zones of antagonism."

Continuing his tests against the lethal and virulent tuberculosis, Schatz was warned to keep his experiments in the university basement. Otherwise, he could risk contamination of the fatal tuberculosis germ throughout the building. Or worse, the entire university. In spite of the danger, Schatz persisted in the basement and was duly rewarded when "zones of antagonism" appeared around the samples of 18-16 and D-1. Meaning, the previously impenetrable tuberculosis bacteria were finally being pushed back. So, not only did Albert Schatz discover an antibiotic effective against gram-negative bacteria, but he also found the first antibiotic known to have activity against the hitherto unassailable tuberculosis.

In mid-October, Albert placed samples of his new antibiotic in a glass tube, sealing the neck with a Bunsen burner, wrapping the tube in cotton wool, and placing it in his pocket. Taking the train from Rutgers to Newark, and then to his parents' house in Passaic, NJ, Albert presented the tube to his mother. He explained to his mother that the odd gift was a new antibiotic that he discovered, which may even kill tuberculosis. Albert Schatz received the only accolade the world would provide—the admiration of his own mother.

Waksman, the Villain

Schatz and Waksman published the discovery, and they filed a patent as co-inventors for the new antibiotic streptomycin. Recognizing the significance of the discovery, Waksman soon moved to diminish Schatz's involvement in the case, referring to him as simply "a pair of hands." Threatening to "kill job chances" in his budding career, Waksman attempted to take all the credit, including financially, academically, and potentially, a looming Nobel from Schatz. A Rutgers University committee eventually awarded Waksman and Schatz 20% of the revenue from the new streptomycin, which was obviously a financial blockbuster for the university. Waksman and Rutgers continued their campaign to intimidate Schatz and to move him from the limelight, not only for financial reasons, but also because of the potential Nobel Prize. Waksman eventually persuaded Schatz to donate his share of the royalties to Rutgers University as a humanitarian gesture. What

Waksman failed to reveal is that he had made his own separate and secretive deal with Rutgers University to receive 20% of the royalties for streptomycin, which over the course of the next five years amounted to $350,000 —over $5 million in 2020.

Rutgers meanwhile collected 2.6 million dollars (almost 40 million dollars in 2020) in streptomycin royalties during the same time period. It would be several years until Schatz learned of this conspiracy and in 1949, he enlisted the services of Attorney Albert Eisenberg, who filed suit against Rutgers University and Waksman. Their main source of evidence: Schatz's detailed notebook. Containing Albert Schatz's meticulous entries of all the actinomyces cultures and subcultures, especially 18-16 and D-1, his notebook was obviously central to the case. But controversy surrounded his journal. The page relating to the critical experiment eleven was clearly and obviously cut from the notebook, allegedly by a Waksman ally. Unfortunately, it was never retrieved. Furthermore, the critical notebook was allegedly obtained by Albert's uncle, Joseph, who supposedly broke into the lab to retrieve it. Controversy swirled around the case.

Suspicion fell immediately upon Waksman. Immediately denouncing the claims, the professor denied any connections between him and the notebook during his deposition by Eisenberg. But Waksman, who had publicly stated he planned to donate his share of the patent money to the university, turned from humanitarian to crook overnight. During his deposition, Selman Waksman admitted to pocketing $350,000 of the 2.6 million in profits received by Rutgers. A public relations disaster was looming not only for Waksman but for Rutgers. A confidential settlement was eventually reached when Rutgers declined to go public in the face of a hostile press. "Rutgers is too smart for its own good," read the headline in the *Passaic Herald News*, Schatz's hometown newspaper.

Nonetheless, although receiving some share of the patent royalties, Schatz's career was over, and his dreams of sharing a Nobel Prize were gone.

Ironically, even cynically, in October 1952, the Nobel Prize Committee awarded the Nobel Prize for Medicine to Waksman for "The Discovery of Streptomycin." *Time* magazine put him on the front cover of their November 7, 1949 edition. Schatz was not mentioned anywhere. His career was over, and his bitterness would follow Albert Schatz to his grave. Despite the lifelong support and commiseration of his friends and family, including Doris Jones, who provided the original chicken samples, Schatz would never recover from the experience. In an interview toward the end of his life about the incident, Schatz broke down and cried. Waksman, for his part, would spend the rest of his career providing long-winded explanations about his primacy in the discovery of streptomycin. In order to silence Doris Jones, and in an attempt to remove the critical importance of her samples, Waksman sent her a $500-check for "flat payment". Doris Jones never cashed the check.

Mankind's search for healing potions predates the eras of Ehrlich, Domagk, Fleming, and Schatz by millennia. In 1962, five Neolithic skeletons were discovered in ancient caves in Europe: two in Spain, two in Belgium, and one in Italy. In these caves, were the remnants of woolly rhinos, Neolithic sheep, reindeer, and mammoth bones. In the small cave in Elsden in Spain, a fossilized Neolithic skull was discovered and minutely examined over the following decades. The hominid had evidence of a dental abscess, clearly a source of great pain. The plaque in "Sid's" teeth was genetically sequenced to shed light on his prehistoric living conditions, diseases, and diet. The results, reported in 2017 in *Nature* [96], showed the DNA sequences of extracts of poplar bark, a primitive form of aspirin. Clearly, Neolithic Sid had been chewing poplar bark, rich in aminosalicylic acid, (modern-day aspirin), as a painkiller. Also, in the same Neolithic plaque, DNA sequences of penicillium mold were found, a primitive form of the antibiotic penicillin. Since penicillium mold tastes nasty and is unpalatable as a food, this was clearly used for medicinal purposes. Millenia before Alexander Fleming reported his 1929 discovery of penicillin, Neolithic Sid was already treating his dental abscess with antibiotics and a painkiller, not too dissimilar to what would be used today. The Neolithic equivalents of aspirin and penicillin had therefore been used 50,000 years before Fleming, ICI, Beecham, Bayer, and Merck ever came along.

Similar archives have been found in Egyptian papyrus 4,000 years ago, including the Ebers papyrus dating to 1550 B.C. This medical papyrus describes the use of willow bark, i.e., aspirin, as an antipyretic and painkiller. A papyrus from 4000 B.C. describes the use of moldy bread, placed in infected wounds in order to treat the infection. Two and a half thousand years ago, Hippocrates in 400 B.C. described the use of the willow bark as a tea to lower fever and reduce pain. Furthermore, the relatively modern Romans were also well aware of the willow bark and its use as a fever-lowering medication and analgesia.

CHAPTER 14

A GLIMMER OF HOPE

In spite of the initial euphoria around the first, and only, antibiotic for tuberculosis, the excitement was short-lived. It became rapidly apparent that the elusive tuberculosis could become resistant to the medication[95]. Just when things are going well, these bacteria find another way to develop resistance to the latest antibiotic. Subsequent research into how the bacterium could develop resistance to streptomycin revealed the bacterium mutated by altering its chromosomal makeup. Even worse, the bacteria could increase its resistance several thousand-fold, which quickly leached into the community. Not only did the bacterium inflict an even more deadly strain into the community, but there was also now no effective cure. At the time, bacteria developing antibiotic resistance was unheard of, let alone studied. This didn't happen with penicillin. So why did it occur with streptomycin? It was back to the drawing board for these scientists. The hunt was on for more effective antibiotics or a combination of antibiotics, which is the mainstay for tuberculosis treatment to this day.

The development of the second anti-tuberculosis drug, Paraminosalicylic acid (PAS), occurred around the same time as

Schatz's discovery of streptomycin[97]. In 1940, Swedish researcher and biochemist Frederick Bernheim decided, by way of random experimentation, to add 1 mg of aspirin (acetylsalicylic acid, or ASA) to a culture of tuberculosis. He found that the concoction increased the metabolic rate of virulent strains of tuberculosis by over 100% compared to the nonvirulent bacteria, which remained in the usual semi-dormant state. Bernheim's first instinct was to use this new discovery as a test to differentiate virulent from nonvirulent strains of TB. Completely overlooking, and not realizing the significance of his findings, Bernheim scribbled his findings on a single sheet of paper, folded it up, and placed it in a small brown envelope, which he mailed to his boss, fellow Swede Jorgen Lehmann.

Describing the events afterward, Lehmann reminisced, "One morning in 1940, I was sitting on my couch in my office at the central laboratory when I received the morning post. There was a small brown envelope from my friend and biochemist and pharmacologist, Frederick Bernheim. In this simple brown envelope, I found a tiny article printed out on just one page. What it said was that if you added 1 mg of salicylic acid (aspirin) to tuberculosis bacteria, you could stimulate oxygen uptake of the bacteria by more than 100%." In the midst of the war against tuberculosis, Lehmann realized the significance of the finding immediately. If a simple molecule of aspirin could accelerate the metabolic rate of virulent tuberculosis, then some chemical modification of that same molecule might throw a spanner in the bacteria's works. If the bacteria could be prevented from replicating, this could potentially create a brand-new antibiotic against tuberculosis. Being distracted by his work on an anticoagulant, it would be three years before Lehmann turned his full attention to modifying the aspirin molecule. The most active derivative turned out to be Paraminosalicylic acid

(PAS), which shut down the tuberculosis bacterium's metabolism to a near standstill. The drug was tested in mice in 1944, and by 1946, 20 patients had been treated successfully. The drug reduced their fevers, the subjects gained weight, and they recovered from consumption. Development of PAS continued to be slow, with the two-drug combination of streptomycin and PAS as a mainstay of treatment for almost ten years.

The next anti-tuberculosis medication to appear, was isoniazid[99]. The molecule itself had been developed as early as 1912, as part of a Ph.D. research program by two Prague research chemists, Hams Meyer and Josef Mally, who were working on the project for their doctorate degrees[99]. Not realizing the significance of the molecules, the chemists' discovery laid dormant for decades. It took another 40 years to discover that the medication had potent antituberculosis activity, including MAP The medication was a derivative of the sulfonamide medication, developed decades earlier by Gerhardt Domagk, who continued his research through the end of World War II. By 1949, 7,000 Germans had been successfully treated for tuberculosis in occupied Germany, unnoticed by the occupying Allied forces.

The new medication was reported to be as effective as PAS, and the possibility of a third anti-TB medication was sensational news. Run by none other than Gerhardt Domagk, the treatment program was missed by the occupying forces until two researchers from Cornell, Walsh McDermott, and Corwin Hinshaw, traveled to West Germany on a "fact-finding" visit and confirmed the sensational finding. No less than three drug companies heard this news from West Berlin and rushed to develop the new antibiotic. These companies were in a heated race to develop and patent the medication. In fact, the patents were filed within just 11 days of each other. Unfortunately for all three companies, the molecule had been identified and reported decades earlier, which invalidated any potential patent. Not to mention it minimized the commercial success of the medication.

By 1942, the medication was ready for clinical trials, and the chosen population was the underserved Navajo Indian Reservation, "Many Farms." In a repeat of the Tuskegee experiment, this hitherto untreated population was suffering an epidemic of tuberculosis and they were considered ideal candidates for a new medicine. This led to the first multidrug treatment of tuberculosis, consisting of isoniazid, streptomycin, and PAS. Although effective, the length of treatment was long—two years to produce remission. Not to mention there was still a high risk for recurrence[95]. Literally, by chance, ethambutol, another dye derivative, was developed by American Cyanamid. In 1946, the company launched a screening program for 5,000 compounds chosen at random, desperate to find a new treatment for TB[100]. Each compound was tested on the usual infected mice, guinea pigs, rabbits, and in vitro via petri dishes, in a bid to identify any molecule with any anti-TB activity. In particular, ethambutol showed activity due to the fact that it existed in two stereoisomers. One isomer, the dextro-isomer, had 12 times the activity as its mirror image. This was a repeat of Pasteur's exponents 100 years earlier. Again capitalizing on any odd and unexplained activity in many thousands of drugs, ethambutol soon replaced PAS on the antibiotic regimen, which reduced the treatment time from two years to 18 months. With Germany occupied by the Allied forces, the next discoveries were left to the other Europeans.

In 1957, researchers were analyzing soil samples from a pine forest in the French Riviera. A hitherto unknown bacteria was isolated and named *Streptococcus meditteraneii*. The researcher, Piero Sensi, discovered its potent antituberculosis activity and called this new generation of antibiotics rifamycin[101,102]. The name was taken from his favorite movie, *Rififi*, a gangster movie of a hapless group of jewel thieves who eventually turned against each other. By 1965, the addition of rifampin to the drug regimen further decreased treatment length to nine months. Importantly, rifampin was found to have potent anti-MAP activity and was to become the first of three potent anti-MAP antibiotics combined in the new "Crohn's antibiotic", RHB-104.

Pyrazinamide, another medication overlooked for decades in the fight against TB, had been identified in pre-World War II Germany when chemists Dalmer and Walter injected vitamin B (nicotinamide) into guinea pigs suffering from tuberculosis[103]. They were astonished when they found that the infected guinea pigs recovered dramatically. Later, they attributed the phenomenon to the benefits of vitamins. But with World War II interceding, development was slow. However, in 1954, the combination of pyrazinamide and isoniazid reported cure rates approaching 90%. Uniquely, pyrazinamide appeared to be able to penetrate tissues so far unassailable by the other medications and began to be recognized as one of the few "sterilizers" of TB. In addition, human duration was now shortened to a record six months, which was incredible given the initial treatment time was 24 months. Two additional drugs would be developed, which would eventually be used in the treatment of MAP.

The second antibiotic used in the anti-MAP cocktail is clofazimine, another offshoot from the dye industry. Developed in Trinity College, Dublin, in 1954[104,105]. Clofazimine, initially known as molecule 0663, is a derivative of a red brick dye, which is a derivative of petroleum. Originally developed as a potential anti-tuberculosis drug, the medication was found to be ineffective against tuberculosis, but had significant activity against leprosy, in many ways a similar bacterium to tuberculosis. Clinical trials in Nigeria in the 1960s demonstrated effectiveness against leprosy[106] and the drug was launched by Novartis in 1969 under the brand name Lamprene. Although ineffective against TB, the medication was tested against MAP, and showed significant success[107]. The medication forms the second of three core antibiotics used in the treatment against MAP[108–110] and in the antibiotic trio to treat Crohn's disease, RHB-104.

The third key antibiotic in the treatment of MAP is clarithromycin[111] (brand name Biaxin). Clarithromycin is a derivative of the parent antibiotic erythromycin, discovered in 1949 by Abelardo Aguilar, a Filipino scientist examining four soil samples in the hopes of a novel antibiotic. In a stroke of luck, a strain of *streptomyces erythreus* was found in the soil samples from the Philippine jungle. The bacteria produced the antibiotic erythromycin, which was then developed by Lilly and launched in 1952. The original brand name was Ilosone, named after the original Philippine region of Iloilo, where it was originally discovered. In 1981, in an attempt to avert GI-upset from erythromycin (nausea, vomiting, and diarrhea), Japanese researchers at Taisho Pharmaceutical modified the original erythromycin module and developed clarithromycin[112]. Touting fewer GI side effects, clarithromycin was approved by the FDA in 1991 and marketed under the brand name Biaxin. The long and unhappy trial of antibiotic boom and bust finally resulted in three medications that were effective against MAP: rifampin, clofazimine and clarithromycin.

A Crohn's Antibiotic

In an attempt to eradicate MAP and reverse GI and systemic complications due to Crohn's, this antibiotic cocktail has been the subject of multiple clinical studies. In 1997, Dr. Gerald Gui[113], a protege of Professor Hermon-Taylor from St George's Hospital, London, was the first to report complete remission in 88.5% of Crohn's symptoms after two years of treatment. This was followed in 2002 by Dr. Ira Shafran[114] from Florida, who showed a sustained improvement in 58.3% of patients after four to 17 months, again using the antibiotic trio. Also, in 2002, Professor Thomas Borody[116] in Sydney, Australia, reported success in 66.6% of patients, which lasted ten years. Three years later, he showed complete clinical endoscopic and biopsy resolution in 32 out of 52 (61.5%) patients examined, and two years later, in 2007, Dr. Thomas Borody[116], again using the same three medications, reported mucosal healing in 22 out of 39 patients, a 56% cure rate. In 2007, Selby et al[115], again in Sydney, Australia, reported very similar results from a prospective randomized double-blind trial, again using rifampin, clarithromycin, and clofazimine for up to three years. At 16 weeks, they reported remission in 66 out of 102 patients (65.7%) compared to 55 out of 111 (49.5%) in the control (untreated) group. This produced impressive statistical significance. These studies created a powerful template for a new medication cocktail combining the same three medications as a treatment, or even a cure, for Crohn's disease.

In 2009, a little-known Israeli biopharmaceutical firm, RedHill Biopharma, located in Tel Aviv partnered with Professor Borody to embark on a new and innovative treatment for Crohn's disease. Recognizing that Crohn's disease is a result of the MAP bacterium, and based on his success with the antibiotic cocktail in treating Crohn's disease, RedHill Biopharma (RBH) and Thomas Borody created RHB-104, the world's first Crohn's disease antibiotic. In December 2020[35], RHB announced the results of its first Phase 3 prospective randomized global trial. The results had an unequivocal success. They enrolled 331 patients with moderate or severe Crohn's disease in the 12-month study. The time since diagnosis of Crohn's disease averaged 10.6 years. The measure of Crohn's disease activity was the Crohn's Disease Activity Index (CDAI), a basket of clinical signs (such as abdominal pain, diarrhea, and general well-being); lab data like complete blood count (CBC), and CRP (an inflammatory marker).

After 26 weeks of treatment, 36.7% of patients in the RHB-104 group had attained clinical remission, i.e., the elusive "cure" as compared with 22.4% of the placebo group, a difference which carried a statistical probability (*p value*) of 0.0048. To put it another way, the odds of this happening by chance was less than one in 200. Similar results were achieved at 52 weeks, when similar, impressive statistical odds (*p value* was 0.0016) were reported, or less than a one in 500 odds of happening by chance. In any clinical trial, a *p value* of less than 0.05 (a one in 20 chance) is considered statistically significant. Therefore, the statistical significance of these studies was undeniable.

In addition, 33 patients also had colonoscopies at the beginning of the trial, and a second colonoscopy at 26 weeks (halfway through the study). At week 26, over five times as many of the RHB-104 patients had achieved endoscopic response compared to the untreated controls. The results were a blockbuster breakthrough in the new paradigm of treating Crohn's disease by using an antibiotic.

The development of RHB-104 was a mixture of inspired genius in the fight against tuberculosis, such as Jorgen Lehmann, who saw the potential of an everyday medicine: aspirin. By transforming this stimulant into an impediment, he outwitted tuberculosis, creating PAS, just in the nick of time to bolster the flailing streptomycin. Others involved "rediscovery" of long-forgotten molecules, which had lain dormant for 30–40 years such as iso-niazid and pyrimidazole. The evidence had always been there, had anybody cared to look. The favored technique to find an elusive cure for tuberculosis was a grueling slugfest by testing hundreds of thousands of molecules in mice, guinea pigs, and petri dishes, in an attempt to identify something, anything, with any activity whatso-ever against the mycobacterium, as was the case with ethambutol.

The fight against MAP and Crohn's disease echoes the long campaign against MAP's great-grandfather, tuberculosis. The similarities between Johne's disease and Crohn's disease were first voiced by Johnathan Dalziel in 1913, over a century ago. In the long and unhappy century that followed, progress has been slow, and skepticism still abounds about the role of MAP in Crohn's disease. The development of the anti-MAP antibiotic RHB-104, and the combination of rifampin, clarithromycin, and clofazimine, promises the first glimmer of hope to effectively treat the actual underlying cause of Crohn's disease, MAP[34].

CHAPTER 15

BEYOND A REASONABLE DOUBT

In most civil legal cases, the evidentiary standard is the "preponderance of the evidence," wherein the plaintiff must present his case to the jury, present the evidence, the witnesses, and provide a convincing argument to the jury. The preponderance of the evidence is usually placed on at least 51% of the evidence substantiating the plaintiff's case. In more serious civil cases, a higher standard of "clear and convincing evidence" is applied. The hurdle in these cases is to prove that their evidence is substantially more likely than not to be true. In criminal cases, a much higher standard is applied—"beyond a reasonable doubt." This is the highest standard of proof in jury trials, and the prosecution must show that their evidence is the only logical explanation available. In other words, no other plausible scenario is possible.

In the case of Crohn's disease, the perpetrator, MAP, is clearly the equivalent of a mass murderer. The evidence of MAP being the perpetrator of Crohn's disease has many levels of circumstantial evidence. Moreover, the recent advent of PCR has brought to light a final piece of the puzzle.

The case against MAP has spanned 150 years and has been an extraordinarily difficult and complex case. At the turn of the 20th century, Crohn's disease was routinely confused with intestinal TB. This case of mistaken identity lasted decades, until 1932 when Crohn finally convinced the medical community that his eponymous disease was a distinct and separate entity, completely different and distinct from intestinal tuberculosis.

For half a decade, circumstantial evidence has abounded in the case against MAP. MAP can be placed at the scene of the crime at multiple sites across the globe. The migratory path taken by migratory birds, principally the starling, coincides exactly with the highest incidence of Johne's disease in cattle and Crohn's disease in man. When starlings were introduced to North America, New Zealand, Australia, and South Africa, to combat crop-destroying grasshoppers, the incidence of Johne's disease in cattle increased. After a few decades, the number of Crohn's disease patients escalated in lockstep.

MAP has been found at the scene of the crime all over the globe. The introduction of the starling into Australia, New Zealand, and South Africa led to a surge in Johne's disease in cattle and a decade later, an explosion of Crohn's disease in the population. The introduction of Johne's-infected cattle to the Czech Republic led directly to a surge in Crohn's disease a few years later[10]. The same scenario played out in Iceland[9] when Johne's-infected sheep were imported in an attempt to mirror the successful sheep industry in their southern neighbor, Scotland. Similar scenarios have played out across the world,

When water runoff from Johne's-infected pasturelands enters the local water supply, MAP can be isolated in local reservoirs and enter the domestic water supplies[67]. This happened when runoff from the Brecon Beacons in South Wales entered the River Taff, resulting in an otherwise unexplainable cluster of Crohn's disease in Cardiff[59], which draws its water supply from the river. Runoff from dairy pastures in Minnesota drains into the Red River which flows north to Winnipeg[7], where the incidence of Crohn's disease is four times higher than their southern US neighbor. unexplained by any theory other than a biological source, in this case, MAP.

More alarmingly, hotpots emerged on individual streets in Winnipeg, where ten individuals from two neighboring families along a single street in Winnipeg developed Crohn's disease within very few years of each other. All the neighbors along this street shared the same waterline. Investigation into this bizarre coincidence revealed MAP in biofilm in the water line supplying the street. MAP has been found in the water supply in multiple communities[67], where the incidence of Crohn's disease spikes is otherwise unexplainable. Crohn's hotspots have been reported in Christchurch New Zealand [79] and Mankato, Minnesota[12], all related to a common and contaminated water supply.

Another line of circumstantial evidence is the genetic transmission of Crohn's disease in individuals with defects in the NOD2 (renamed to CARD15) gene. This gene codes for intestinal defense against pathogens such as MAP. Since this gene is transmitted from generation to generation, it should be no surprise that Crohn's disease is likely transmitted down generational lines. The finding of MAP bacteria in the breastmilk of patients with Crohn's disease provides the damning link between Crohn's and its hereditary transmission. The nursing mother with Crohn's unknowingly transmits MAP to her similarly genetically susceptible newborns, unwittingly transmitting the bacteria in her own breast milk. Not surprisingly, the incidence of Crohn's disease in identical twins is extremely high, as a result of ingesting MAP disease in their mother's milk.

In our imaginary criminal trial, the defense team had piles and piles of evidence rejecting the connection between MAP and Crohn's in the late 20th century. I'll admit, it was pretty convincing. The MAP bacteria could not be identified by microscopy in Crohn's disease tissue, nor could it be cultured in conventional culture mediums. There was no smoking gun. The glove didn't fit. This was convincing evidence against the role of MAP in the causation of Crohn's disease. We now know MAP, like its great-grandfather tuberculosis, is extremely difficult to identify in tissue biopsies because of its thick, waxy coat, and is extraordinarily difficult to culture. Specifically, it requires specific culture media, temperature, and culture conditions. Even then, it may take months for the bacteria finally to be identified.

The balance of the evidence tipped in 1989 when Rodrick Chiodini took samples of Crohn's disease tissue from a young patient, (the "Linda" cultures) and fed extracts from these samples to young goats, who eventually developed intestinal changes of Crohn's disease[25]. Similar experiments were confirmed in other animal models.

A Smoking Gun

It was not until PCR became widely available that MAP was identified as the culprit all along. PCR was able to identify MAP's genetic fingerprints in samples of Crohn's disease tissues. The presence of MAP's DNA at the crime scene, like any *CSI* episode, provided incontrovertible evidence of MAP's guilt. When researchers examined the tissues from both old and new cases, IS900, the genetic fingerprint of MAP, was identified in practically all the tissues examined.

Chiodini again provided the missing link. He demonstrated that MAP could shed its protective coat and become a spheroplast, an invisible "ghost" of MAP undetectable by conventional microscopy. The spheroplast, barely more than a tangle of DNA and essential organelles, enters its victim's cells which provide nutrition, oxygen, and shelter from the victim's marauding immune system circulating outside. MAP was not only an elusive perpetrator, impossible to identify by conventional microscopy, but was a master of disguise, by shedding its outer cell wall to become invisible.

Finally, MAP had been positively identified, and the cold case was solved. Given this evidence, and especially the presence of the smoking gun IS900, the evidence is convincing, overwhelming, and proves beyond all reasonable doubt the role of MAP in Crohn's disease. The evidence was irrefutable and undeniable.

However, skeptics still remain. The identification of MAP in over-the-counter milk products and infant formula[2] triggered a public panic both in Europe and the US. Rightfully so. But the US Department of Agriculture, desiring to protect the politically influential dairy lobby, denied any association between MAP and Crohn's disease. They even went as far as to refuse to create their own studies to verify this link. Other government agencies, like the CDC, are reluctant to break ranks, therefore, federal research dollars have been withheld from further research. The medical community, even seasoned gastroenterologists and surgeons, have not heard of the role of MAP in Crohn's disease. Unfortunately, the public is unaware.

Eradicating MAP
The campaign to eradicate MAP must follow the same campaign implemented a century ago to eradicate bovine tuberculosis from the cattle herds of Europe and America. Mandatory screening of

dairy herds, screening of milk and dairy products, and pasteurization of milk eliminated intestinal tuberculosis. Bovine tuberculosis was uniquely susceptible to pasteurization, practically eliminating intestinal tuberculosis from contaminated milk. Unfortunately, the unique resistance of MAP to pasteurization makes this same plan infinitely more difficult.

Intensive screening of dairy herds and milk products for MAP is available, but less rigorously implemented than those for tuberculosis. It can, however, be successful, and is implemented in the more modern robot dairy herds, including that of my cousin Robert Armstrong, who operates one of the largest robotic dairy farms in Europe, where the process of milk production is efficient, safe, and cost-effective compared to conventional milk production. The entire process is computer-driven. Enticed by a constant supply of fodder, individual cows enter a milking stall, where sensors identify the individual cow, laser sensors map out the cow's udder, and spray the teats with disinfectant. Guided again by lasers, milking "cups" are robotically placed on each of the four teats, and the milking process begins. The cows enjoy the milking process, are more than content to chew the readily available fodder, and even compete with each other to enter the next available milking stall. Milk output is closely monitored by a remote computer, and when each "udder" has been adequately milked, the milking cups automatically disengage, and the cow strolls out of the stall, making room for the next. Cows enter the stalls many times a day, often on six or eight occasions, night and day. Monitoring the process is efficient, hygienic, and safe. The milk itself is routinely analyzed for MAP, bovine TB, and other pathogens. The process is incredible to witness and is the future of milk production, but possible only at enormous capital expenditure. Unfortunately, it is too early to see a real drop in Crohn's disease, but it is coming in time.

One way to stop the spread of MAP through the milk supply would be to eradicate the vector of the bacteria, i.e., the "avian" transmitter, likely the starling. But how do we get rid of an entire species of bird, even though they are the greatest winged pests throughout the world? Given they are an endemic pest in every continent, this would be an impossible task. Before anyone gets carried away, the first step would be to perform more research into the role of the starling in spreading MAP. A 2005 publication in *Applied and Environmental Microbiology* [66] tested several species of birds and mammals in nine dairy farms in Wisconsin and Georgia for MAP: 774 animals representing 25 mammalians and 22 avian species were collected, including the starling, sparrow, armadillo, gopher, raccoon, and skunk, amongst others. The study reported MAP was found in each starling examined. The bad news was only seven starlings were tested, and MAP was also found in many other animals tested. Even if the bird vector were controlled, the vast majority of MAP is not in the bird population, but in Johne's-infected dairy herds, the vast "reservoir" of disease, where MAP is transmitted from cow to cow. The importance of monitoring, regulating—and even potentially licensing—dairy farms for MAP surveillance in known high-risk locations, such as slurry pits[117] and liquid manure spreaders may provide some degree of control. Screening for MAP in dairy cows and early culling of Johne's-infected cattle would go a long way in at least diminishing the problem, even though it may never completely eliminate it[117].

Given the global scale of MAP contamination, the starling is the only plausible vector of MAP. Migrating swarms of starlings count in the tens or hundreds of thousands of birds, which literally blacken the sky as they spew their contaminated dropping over pastures, grazing lands, and cattle feeders in Europe, America, Australia, New Zealand, and South Africa. The other avian and mammalian suspects have alibis. Sparrows are solitary birds, incapable of inflicting this damage. Armadillos or gophers in Europe, America, Australia, and New Zealand live underground and have little contact with dairy cattle. However, since this evidence is based only on a few starlings, it is obvious that much research is needed.

Reports have emerged in the press of starlings "dropping dead out of the skies" as local farmers take it upon themselves to place poison around their cattle feeders to rid themselves of this predatory pest. Broadcasting recordings of the starling's distress call have been attempted, apparently with some success. Destruction of nesting habitats has been proposed. In a politically charged and conservation-minded world, none of these methods will be found acceptable.

To those cases which have fallen through the safety nets, the vaccination for Crohn's disease is left to a single individual, Dr. Herman Taylor, who single-handedly is developing an anti-MAP vaccine for use in patients with Crohn's toward its prevention. The vaccine is promoted through his website www.HAV-vaccine.com, where individual investors are solicited. Not only was the vaccine intended as a preventative measure, but it also was designed to cure people who currently have Crohn's. Lacking any government research dollars, this barebones effort, in conjunction with the Jenner Institute of the University of Oxford, is in its very early stages, and the vaccine, if it works, will be many years away. The development of an antibiotic cocktail against MAP has shown dramatic success in treating Crohn's disease. Developed by an Israeli company, RedHill Biopharma, without any government backing and conducted entirely through the private sector, this dramatically effective antibiotic is a rare glimmer of hope in the battle against Crohn's disease[35].

The cure for Crohn's has taken many decades to arrive at after the conclusion that both Johne's and Crohn's disease are one and the same. Both are caused by MAP and both are zoonoses, transmitted from birds to cows as Johne's disease and ultimately to man, as Crohn's disease. We no longer need to label Crohn's disease as an "idiopathic" disease or use "empiric" treatments such as steroids. The mold has been broken. We now have the first of a kind, direct, and targeted treatment of a bacterial disease with a specific, effective antibiotic cocktail. This is the first of a new antibiotic treatment regimen, but it will not be the last. What is more important is the recognition that Crohn's disease is a zoonotic bacterial infection and can be treated with a new and evolving paradigm of antibiotic regimens to achieve the ultimate goal—a cure for Crohn's.

BIBLIOGRAPHY

1. Taylor TK, Wilks CR, McQueen DS. Isolation of Mycobacterium paratuberculosis from the milk of a cow with Johne's disease. *Veterinary Record*. 1981;109(24). doi:10.1136/vr.109.24.532

2. Acharya KR, Dhand NK, Whittington RJ, Plain KM. Detection of Mycobacterium avium subspecies paratuberculosis in powdered infant formula using IS900 quantitative PCR and liquid culture media. *International Journal of Food Microbiology*. 2017;257. doi:10.1016/j.ijfoodmicro.2017.06.005

3. Naser SA, Schwartz D, Shafran I. Isolation of Mycobacterium avium subsp paratuberculosis from breast milk of Crohn's disease patients. *The American Journal of Gastroenterology*. 2000;95(4). doi:10.1111/j.1572-0241.2000.01954.x

4. Hermon-Taylor J. Mycobacterium avium subspecies paratuberculosis is a cause of Crohn's disease. *Gut*. 2001;49(6). doi:10.1136/gut.49.6.755

5. Sechi LA, Dow CT. Mycobacterium avium ss. paratuberculosis Zoonosis - The Hundred Year War - Beyond Crohn's

Disease. *Frontiers in Immunology.* 2015;6(MAR). doi:10.3389/fimmu.2015.00096

6. Collins FM. Mycobacterial pathogenesis: a historical perspective. *Frontiers in bioscience : a journal and virtual library.* 1998;3. doi:10.2741/A285

7. Hermon-Taylor J. Mycobacterium avium subspecies paratuberculosis, Crohn's disease and the Doomsday scenario. *Gut Pathogens.* 2009;1(1). doi:10.1186/1757-4749-1-15

8. Phavichitr N, Cameron DJS, Catto-Smith AG. Increasing incidence of Crohn's disease in Victorian children. *Journal of Gastroenterology and Hepatology (Australia).* 2003;18(3). doi:10.1046/j.1440-1746.2003.02975.x

9. Agnarsson Ú, Björnsson S, Jóhansson JH, Sigurdsson L. Inflammatory bowel disease in Icelandic children 1951-2010. Population-based study involving one nation over six decades. *Scandinavian Journal of Gastroenterology.* 2013;48(12). doi:10.3109/00365521.2013.845799

10. Schwarz J, Sýkora J, Cvalínová D, et al. Inflammatory bowel disease incidence in Czech children: A regional prospective study, 2000-2015. *World Journal of Gastroenterology.* 2017;23(22). doi:10.3748/wjg.v23.i22.4090

11. Kruiningen HJV, Colombel JF, Cartun RW, et al. An in-depth study of Crohn's disease in two French families. *Gastroenterology.* 1993;104(2). doi:10.1016/0016-5085(93)90401-W

12. Lawrance IC, Maxwell L, Doe W. A clustering of Crohn's disease in Mankato, Minnesota. *Inflammatory Bowel Diseases.* 2001;7(1). doi:10.1097/00054725-200102000-00004

13. Harris NB, Barletta RG. Mycobacterium avium subsp. paratuberculosis in Veterinary Medicine. *Clinical Microbiology Reviews.* 2001;14(3). doi:10.1128/CMR.14.3.489-512.2001

14. O'Reilly CE, O'Connor L, Anderson W, et al. Surveillance of bulk raw and commercially pasteurized cows' milk from approved Irish liquid-milk pasteurization plants to determine the incidence of Mycobacterium paratuberculosis. *Applied and Environmental Microbiology.* 2004;70(9). doi:10.1128/AEM.70.9.5138-5144.2004

15. Millar D, Ford J, Sanderson J, et al. IS900 PCR to detect Mycobacterium paratuberculosis in retail supplies of whole pasteurized cows' milk in England and Wales. *Applied and Environmental Microbiology.* 1996;62(9). doi:10.1128/aem.62.9.3446-3452.1996

16. Rathnaiah G, Zinniel DK, Bannantine JP, et al. Pathogenesis, molecular genetics, and genomics of Mycobacterium avium subsp. paratuberculosis, the etiologic agent of Johne's disease. *Frontiers in Veterinary Science.* 2017;4(NOV). doi:10.3389/fvets.2017.00187

17. Collins MT. Mycobacterium paratuberculosis: A Potential Food-Borne Pathogen? *Journal of Dairy Science.* 1997;80(12). doi:10.3168/jds.S0022-0302(97)76321-5

18. Chiodini RJ, van Kruiningen HJ, Thayer WR, Coutu JA. Spheroplastic phase of mycobacteria isolated from patients with Crohn's disease. *Journal of Clinical Microbiology.* 1986;24(3). doi:10.1128/jcm.24.3.357-363.1986

19. Hermon-Taylor J, Bull TJ, Sheridan JM, Cheng J, Stellakis ML, Sumar N. Causation of Crohn's disease by Mycobacterium avium subspecies paratuberculosis. *Canadian Journal of Gastroenterology.* 2000;14(6). doi:10.1155/2000/798305

20. Thompson DE. The role of mycobacteria in Crohn's disease. *Journal of Medical Microbiology.* 1994;41(2). doi:10.1099/00222615-41-2-74

21. Su HY, Gupta V, Day AS, Gearry RB. Rising Incidence of Inflammatory Bowel Disease in Canterbury, New Zealand. *Inflammatory Bowel Diseases.* 2016;22(9). doi:10.1097/MIB.0000000000000829

22. Economou M, Pappas G. New global map of Crohn's disease: Genetic, environmental, and socioeconomic correlations. *Inflammatory Bowel Diseases.* 2008;14(5). doi:10.1002/ibd.20352

23. M 'koma AE. Clinical Medicine insights: Gastroenterology Inflammatory Bowel Disease: An Expanding Global Health Problem. *Clinical Medicine Insights: Gastroenterology.* 2013;6.

24. Alatab S, Sepanlou SG, Ikuta K, et al. The global, regional, and national burden of inflammatory bowel disease in 195 countries and territories, 1990–2017: a systematic analysis for the Global Burden of Disease Study 2017. *The*

Lancet Gastroenterology & Hepatology. 2020;5(1). doi:10.1016/ S2468-1253(19)30333-4

25. van Kruiningen HJ, Chiodini RJ, Thayer WR, Coutu JA, Merkal RS, Runnels PL. Experimental disease in infant goats induced by a Mycobacterium isolated from a patient with Crohn's disease - A preliminary report. *Digestive Diseases and Sciences.* 1986;31(12). doi:10.1007/BF01299814

26. Moss MT, Green EP, Tizard ML, Malik ZP, Hermon-Taylor J. Specific detection of Mycobacterium paratuberculosis by DNA hybridisation with a fragment of the insertion element IS900. *Gut.* 1991;32(4). doi:10.1136/gut.32.4.395

27. Autschbach F, Eisold S, Hinz U, et al. High prevalence of Mycobacterium avium subspecies paratuberculosis IS900 DNA in gut tissues from individuals with Crohn's disease. *Gut.* 2005;54(7). doi:10.1136/gut.2004.045526

28. Hermon-Taylor J. Mycobacterium avium subspecies paratuberculosis in the causation of Crohn's disease. *World Journal of Gastroenterology.* 2000;6(5). doi:10.3748/wjg.v6.i5.630

29. Bannantine JP, Li L, Mwangi M, Cote R, Raygoza Garay JA, Kapur V. Complete Genome Sequence of Mycobacterium avium subsp. paratuberculosis, Isolated from Human Breast Milk. *Genome Announcements.* 2014;2(1). doi:10.1128/ genomea.01252-13

30. Chiodini RJ, Chamberlin WM, Sarosiek J, McCallum RW. Crohn's disease and the mycobacterioses: A quarter century

later. Causation or simple association? *Critical Reviews in Microbiology*. 2012;38(1). doi:10.3109/1040841X.2011.638273

31. Slana I, Paolicchi F, Janstova B, Navratilova P, Pavlik I. Detection methods for Mycobacterium avium subsp. paratuberculosis in milk and milk products: A review. *Veterinarni Medicina*. 2008;53(6). doi:10.17221/1859-VETMED

32. Sartor RB. Does Mycobacterium avium subspecies paratuberculosis cause Crohn's disease? *Gut*. 2005;54(7). doi:10.1136/gut.2004.055889

33. European Commission. Directorate-General Health and Consumer Protection. Possible links between Crohn's disease and MAP. *Report of the scientific committee on animal health and animal welfare*. Published online March 21, 2000.

34. Borody TJ, Leis S, Warren EF, Surace R. Treatment of severe Crohn's disease using antimycobacterial triple therapy - Approaching a cure? *Digestive and Liver Disease*. 2002;34(1). doi:10.1016/S1590-8658(02)80056-1

35. RedHills Biopharma. Efficacy and Safety of Anti-MAP Therapy in Adult Crohn's Disease (MAPUS). www.clinical trails.gov

36. Kuenstner JT, Naser S, Chamberlin W, et al. The consensus from the Mycobacterium avium ssp. paratuberculosis (MAP) conference 2017. *Frontiers in Public Health*. 2017;5. doi:10.3389/fpubh.2017.00208

37. Barnes DS. Historical perspective on the etiology of tuberculosis. *Microbes and Infection.* 2000;2(4). doi:10.1016/S1286-4579(00)00323-3

38. Cambau E, Drancourt M. Steps towards the discovery of Mycobacterium tuberculosis by Robert Koch, 1882. *Clinical Microbiology and Infection.* 2014;20(3). doi:10.1111/1469-0691.12555

39. Sakula A. Robert Koch: Centenary of the discovery of the tubercle bacillus, 1882. *Thorax.* 1982;37(4). doi:10.1136/thx.37.4.246

40. Brock T.D. The Etiology of Tuberculosis. *The American Journal of the Medical Sciences.* 1882;84(167). doi:10.1097/00000441-188207000-00050

41. Koch R. The Etiology of Tuberculosis. *Reviews of Infectious Diseases.* 1982;4(6). doi:10.1093/clinids/4.6.1270

42. Candler C. The Etiology of Tuberculosis. *The Lancet.* 1891;138 (3551). DOI:10.1016/S0140-6736(01)75977-6

43. Kaplan L. THE DOCTOR'S WORLD; Revisionist History Sees Pasteur As Liar Who Stole Rival's Ideas. Published online 1995.

44. The lübeck catastrophe. *British Medical Journal.* 1931;1(3674). doi:10.1136/bmj.1.3674.986

45. Report on the lübeck disaster. *The Lancet.* 1930;215(5571). doi:10.1016/S0140-6736(00)70979-2

46. Fox GJ, Orlova M, Schurr E. Tuberculosis in Newborns: The Lessons of the "Lübeck Disaster" (1929–1933). *PLoS Pathogens.* 2016;12(1). doi:10.1371/journal.ppat.1005271

47. Editorial. The Lubeck catastrophe. *The British Medical Journal.* Published online June 6, 1931:986-988.

48. Anon. Judge commits suicide. *The Melbourne Argus.* August 1932.

49. Twort FW, Ingram LY. Some Further Researches on Johne's Disease. *The Veterinary Journal (1900).* 1912;68(10). doi:10.1016/s0372-5545(17)65885-1

50. Coss S. *The FEVER of 1721.* Simon & Schuster; 2016.

51. Dalziel TK. Thomas Kennedy Dalziel 1861-1924. Chronic interstitial enteritis. *Diseases of the colon and rectum.* 1989;32(12). doi:10.1007/BF02553886

52. Crohn BB, Ginzburg L, Oppenheimer GD. Regional ileitis: A pathologic and clinical entity. *Journal of the American Medical Association.* 1932;99(16). doi:10.1001/jama.1932.02740680019005

53. Ginzburg l, Oppenheimer GD. Non-specific granulomata of the intestines. *Annals of surgery.* 1933;98(6). DOI:10.1097/00000658-193312000-00008

54. Green EP, Tizard MLV, Moss MT, et al. Sequence and character-istics of IS900, an insertion element identified in a human Crohn's disease isolate of Mycobacterium paratuberculosis. *Nucleic Acids Research.* 1989;17(22):9063-9073. doi:10.1093/nar/17.22.9063

55. Fredricks DN, Relman DA. Sequence-based identification of microbial pathogens: A reconsideration of Koch's postulates. *Clinical Microbiology Reviews.* 1996;9(1). doi:10.1128/cmr.9.1.18-33.1996

56. Pickup RW, Rhodes G, Hermon-Taylor J. Mycobacterium avium subspecies paratuberculosis, Johne's disease and Crohn's disease. In: *Environmental Medicine.* ; 2010.

57. Jabandziev P, Pinkasova T, Kunovsky L, et al. Regional Incidence of Inflammatory Bowel Disease in a Czech Pediatric Population: 16 Years of Experience (2002-2017). *Journal of pediatric gastroenterology and nutrition.* 2020;70(5). doi:10.1097/MPG.0000000000002660

58. Rose JDR, Roberts GM, Williams G, Mayberry JF, Rhodes J. Cardiff Crohn's disease jubilee: The incidence over 50 years. *Gut.* 1988;29(3). doi:10.1136/gut.29.3.346

59. Mayberry JF, Hitchens RAN. Distribution of Crohn's disease in Cardiff. *Social Science and Medicine Part C Medical Geography.* 1978;12(2). doi:10.1016/0160-8002(78)90018-7

60. Gearry RB, Chb MB, Richardson A, et al. High Incidence of Crohn's Disease in Canterbury, New Zealand : Results of an Epidemiologic Study. *Inflammatory Bowel Diseases.* 2006;12(10).

61. Gunesh S, Thomas GAO, Williams GT, Roberts A, Hawthorne AB. The incidence of Crohn's disease in Cardiff over the last 75 years: An update for 1996-2005. *Alimentary Pharmacology and Therapeutics*. 2008;27(3). doi:10.1111/j.1365-2036.2007.03576.x

62. Hellers G. Crohn's disease in Stockholm County 1955-1974. *Acta Chirurgica Scandinavica*. 1979;145(Suppl. 490).

63. Wolf R, Barkema HW, de Buck J, et al. High herd-level prevalence of Mycobacterium avium subspecies paratuberculosis in Western Canadian dairy farms, based on environmental sampling. *Journal of Dairy Science*. 2014;97(10). doi:10.3168/jds.2014-8101

64. Grant IR, Ball HJ, Rowe MT. Incidence of Mycobacterium paratuberculosis in bulk raw and commercially pasteurized cows' milk from approved dairy processing establishments in the United Kingdom. *Applied and Environmental Microbiology*. 2002;68(5). doi:10.1128/AEM.68.5.2428-2435.2002

65. Ellingson JLE, Anderson JL, Koziczkowski JJ, et al. Detection of viable Mycobacterium avium subsp. paratuberculosis in retail pasteurized whole milk by two culture methods and PCR. *Journal of Food Protection*. 2005;68(5). doi:10.4315/0362-028X-68.5.966

66. Corn JL, Manning EJB, Sreevatsan S, Fischer JR. Isolation of Mycobacterium avium subsp. paratuberculosis from free-ranging birds and mammals on livestock premises. *Applied*

and Environmental Microbiology. 2005;71(11). doi:10.1128/AEM.71.11.6963-6967.2005

67. Falkinham JO. Mycobacterium avium complex (Mac) in water distribution systems and household plumbing in the united states. *Water (Switzerland).* 2020;12(12). doi:10.3390/w12123338

68. Lombard JE, Wagner BA, Smith RL, et al. Evaluation of environmental sampling and culture to determine Mycobacterium avium subspecies paratuberculosis distribution and herd infection status on US dairy operations. *Journal of Dairy Science.* 2006;89(11). doi:10.3168/jds.S0022-0302(06)72461-4

69. Lopez RN, Evans HM, Appleton L, et al. Point Prevalence of Pediatric Inflammatory Bowel Disease in New Zealand in 2015: Initial Results from the PINZ Study. *Inflammatory Bowel Diseases.* 2017;23(8). doi:10.1097/MIB.0000000000001138

70. Sung N, Collins MT. Thermal tolerance of Mycobacterium paratuberculosis. *Applied and Environmental Microbiology.* 1998;64(3). doi:10.1128/aem.64.3.999-1005.1998

71. Sung NM, Kaspar CW, Collins MT. *Determination of D-Values in Studies on the Thermal Tolerance of Mycobacterium Paratuberculosis.*; 1997.

72. Chiodini RJ, Hermon-Taylor J. The thermal resistance of Mycobacterium paratuberculosis in raw milk under conditions simulating pasteurization. *Journal of Veterinary Diagnostic Investigation.* 1993;5(4). doi:10.1177/104063879300500424

73. Stabel JR. Johne's disease and milk: Do consumers need to worry? In: *Journal of Dairy Science*. Vol 83. ; 2000. doi:10.3168/jds.S0022-0302(00)75034-X

74. Grant IR, Stabel JR. Does Mycobacterium paratuberculosis survive current pasteurization conditions? (multiple letters). *Applied and Environmental Microbiology*. 1998;64(7). doi:10.1128/AEM.64.7.2760-2761.1998

75. Greger M. Paratuberculosis And Crohn's Disease: Got Milk?www.mad-cow.org › paraTB.

76. Chamberlin W, Borody T, Naser S. MAP-associated Crohn's Disease. MAP, Koch's postulates, causality, and Crohn's Disease. *Digestive and Liver Disease*. 2007;39(8). doi:10.1016/j.dld.2007.05.012

77. M'Koma AE. Inflammatory bowel disease: An expanding global health problem. *Clinical Medicine Insights: Gastroenterology*. 2013;6. doi:10.4137/CGast.S12731

78. Ng S, Shi H, Hamidi N. Worldwide incidence and prevalence of inflammatory bowel disease in the 21ˢᵗ century: A systematic review of population-based studies. *The Lancet*. 2017;390(10114).

79. Gearry RB, Richardson A, Frampton CMA, et al. High incidence of Crohn's disease in Canterbury, New Zealand: Results of an epidemiologic study. *Inflammatory Bowel Diseases*. 2006;12(10). doi:10.1097/01.mib.0000231572.88806.b9

80. Linz GM, Homan HJ, Gaulker SM, Penry LB, Bleier WJ. European Starlings : a Review of an Invasive Species With

Far-Reaching Impacts. *Managing Vertebrate Invasive Species: Proceedings of an International Symposium.* 2007;1942.

81. Ogura Y, Bonen DK, Inohara N, et al. A frameshift mutation in NOD2 associated with susceptibility to Crohn's disease. *Nature.* 2001;411(6837). doi:10.1038/35079114

82. Hugot JP, Chamaillard M, Zouali H, et al. Association of NOD2 leucine-rich repeat variants with susceptibility to Crohn's disease. *Nature.* 2001;411(6837). doi:10.1038/35079107

83. Colombel JF. The CARD15 (also known as NOD2) gene in Crohn's disease: Are there implications for current clinical practice? *Clinical Gastroenterology and Hepatology.* 2003;1(1). doi:10.1053/jcgh.2003.50002

84. Hisamatsu T, Suzuki M, Reinecker HC, Nadeau WJ, McCormick BA, Podolsky DK. CARD15/NOD2 functions as an antibacterial factor in human intestinal epithelial cells. *Gastroenterology.* 2003;124(4). doi:10.1053/gast.2003.50153

85. Cho JH. The Nod2 gene in Crohn's disease: Implications for future research into the genetics and immunology of Crohn's disease. *Inflammatory Bowel Diseases.* 2001;7(3). doi:10.1097/00054725-200108000-00014

86. Büning C, Genschel J, Bühner S, et al. Mutations in the NOD2/CARD15 gene in Crohn's disease are associated with ileocecal resection and are a risk factor for reoperation. *Alimentary Pharmacology and Therapeutics.* 2004;19(10). doi:10.1111/j.1365-2036.2004.01967.x

87. Duclos B, Dupas JL, Galmiche JP, et al. A frameshift mutation in NOD2 associated with susceptibility to Crohn's disease. *Nature*. 2001;411(May).

88. Bull TJ, Gilbert SC, Sridhar S, et al. A novel multi-antigen virally vectored vaccine against Mycobacterium avium subspecies paratuberculosis. *PLoS ONE*. 2007;2(11). doi:10.1371/journal.pone.0001229

89. Volz A, Sutter G. Modified Vaccinia Virus Ankara: History, Value in Basic Research, and Current Perspectives for Vaccine Development. In: *Advances in Virus Research*. Vol 97. ; 2017. doi:10.1016/bs.aivir.2016.07.001

90. Sutter G. A vital gene for modified vaccinia virus Ankara replication in human cells. *Proceedings of the National Academy of Sciences of the United States of America*. 2020;117(12). doi:10.1073/pnas.2001335117

91. Folegatti PM, Ewer KJ, Aley PK, et al. Safety and immunogenicity of the ChAdOx1 nCoV-19 vaccine against SARS-CoV-2: a preliminary report of a phase 1/2, single-blind, randomized controlled trial. *The Lancet*. 2020;396(10249). doi:10.1016/S0140-6736(20)31604-4

92. Pringle P. *Experiment Eleven: Dark Secrets behind the Discovery of a Wonderdrug*. Bloomsbury; 2012.

93. Zaffiri L, Gardner J, Toledo-Pereyra LH. History of antibiotics. from salvarsan to cephalosporins. *Journal of*

Investigative Surgery. 2012;25(2). doi:10.3109/08941939.2012 .664099

94. Fleming A. On the antibacterial action of cultures of penicillium, with special reference to their use in the isolation of B. influenzae. 1929. *Bulletin of the World Health Organization*. 2001;79(8). doi:10.1093/clinids/2.1.129

95. Murray JF, Schraufnagel DE, Hopewell PC. Treatment of tuberculosis: A historical perspective. *Annals of the American Thoracic Society*. 2015;12(12). doi:10.1513/ AnnalsATS.201509-632PS

96. Weyrich LS, Duchene S, Soubrier J, et al. Neanderthal behavior, diet, and disease inferred from ancient DNA in dental calculus. *Nature*. 2017;544(7650). doi:10.1038/nature21674

97. Lehmann J. Twenty years afterward: historical notes on the discovery of the antituberculosis effect of para-aminosalicylic acid (PAS) and the first clinical trials. *American Review of Respiratory Disease, 90(6), pp 953–95*. Published online 1964.

98. Riva MA. From milk to rifampicin and back again: History of failures and successes in the treatment for tuberculosis. *Journal of Antibiotics*. 2014;67(9). doi:10.1038/ja.2014.108

99. Heysell S, Mpgama S. Re-evaluating the role of isoniazid in treatment of pulmonary tuberculosis. *The Lancet Microbe*. 2020;1(2). doi:10.1016/s2666-5247(20)30034-3

100. Shepherd RG, Baughn C, Cantrall Ml, Goodstein B, Thomas JP, Wilkinson RG. Structure-Activity Studies Leading to Ethambutol, A New Type of Antituberculous Compound. *Annals Of The New York Academy of Sciences.* 1966;135(2). DOI:10.1111/J.1749-6632.1966.TB45516.X

101. Asif M. Rifampin and Their Analogs: A Development of Antitubercular Drugs. *World Journal of Organic Chemistry.* 2013;1(2).

102. Sensi P. History of the development of rifampin. *Reviews of Infectious Diseases.* 1983;5. doi:10.1093/clinids/5. Supplement_3.S402

103. Zhang Y, Shi W, Zhang W, Mitchison D. Mechanisms of Pyrazinamide Action and Resistance. *Microbiology Spectrum.* 2014;2(4). doi:10.1128/microbiolspec.mgm2-0023-2013

104. Lu Y, Zheng MQ, Wang B, et al. Activities of clofazimine against Mycobacterium tuberculosis in vitro and in vivo. *Zhonghua jie he he hu xi za zhi = Zhonghua jiehe he huxi zazhi = Chinese journal of tuberculosis and respiratory diseases.* 2008;31(10).

105. Jagannath C, Reddy MV, Kailasam S, O'Sullivan JF, Gangadharam PRJ. Chemotherapeutic activity of clofazimine and its analogues against Mycobacterium tuberculosis: In vitro, intracellular, and in vivo studies. *American Journal of Respiratory and Critical Care Medicine.* 1995;151(4). doi:10.1164/ajrccm.151.4.7697235

106. Garrelts JC. Clofazimine: A review of its use in leprosy and Mycobacterium avium complex

infection. *DICP, Annals of Pharmacotherapy.* 1991;25(5). doi:10.1177/106002809102500513

107. Hermon-Taylor J. Treatment with drugs active against Mycobacterium avium subspecies paratuberculosis can heal Crohn's disease: More evidence for a neglected public health tragedy. *Digestive and Liver Disease.* 2002;34(1). doi:10.1016/S1590-8658(02)80052-4

108. Lal S, Steinhart AH. Antibiotic therapy for Crohn's disease: A review. *Canadian Journal of Gastroenterology.* 2006;20(10). doi:10.1155/2006/250490

109. Card T, Logan RFA, Rodrigues LC, Wheeler JG. Antibiotic use and the development of Crohn's disease. *Gut.* 2004;53(2). doi:10.1136/gut.2003.025239

110. Hviid A, Svanström H, Frisch M. Antibiotic use and inflammatory bowel diseases in childhood. *Gut.* 2011;60(1). doi:10.1136/gut.2010.219683

111. Alvarez-Elcoro S, Enzler MJ. The macrolides: Erythromycin, clarithromycin, and azithromycin. In: *Mayo Clinic Proceedings.* Vol 74. ; 1999. doi:10.4065/74.6.613

112. Amsden GW. Erythromycin, clarithromycin, and azithromycin: Are the differences real? *Clinical Therapeutics.* 1996;18(1). doi:10.1016/S0149-2918(96)80179-2

113. Gui GPH, Thomas PRS, Tizard MLV, Lake J, Sanderson JD, Hermon-Taylor J. Two-year-outcomes analysis of Crohn's

disease treated with rifabutin and macrolide antibiotics. *Journal of Antimicrobial Chemotherapy.* 1997;39(3). doi:10.1093/jac/39.3.393

114. Shafran I, Kugler L, El-Zaatari FAK, Naser SA, Sandoval J. Open clinical trial of rifabutin and clarithromycin therapy in Crohn's disease. *Digestive and Liver Disease.* 2002;34(1). doi:10.1016/S1590-8658(02)80055-X

115. Selby W, Pavli P, Crotty B, et al. Two-Year Combination Antibiotic Therapy With Clarithromycin, Rifabutin, and Clofazimine for Crohn's Disease. *Gastroenterology.* 2007;132(7). doi:10.1053/j.gastro.2007.03.031

116. Borody TJ, Bilkey S, Wettstein AR, Leis S, Pang G, Tye S. Anti-mycobacterial therapy in Crohn's disease heals mucosa with longitudinal scars. *Digestive and Liver Disease.* 2007;39(5). doi:10.1016/j.dld.2007.01.008

117. Schukken YH, Mitchell RM, Pradhan AK, et al. Elimination of Mycobacterium avium subspecies paratuberculosis from dairy farms: fact or fiction? In: *Proceedings of the 10th International Colloquium on Paratuberculosis, Minneapolis, Minnesota, USA, 9-14 August 2009.* International Association for Paratuberculosis; 2009:109-113. Accessed March 10, 2015. http://cabdirect. org/abstracts/20123141245.html

BLURB

A *Cure for Crohn's* is a true life medical mystery of how the cause of a disease which affects 1.5 million Americans, mostly adolescents, has been kept undercover from the public.

An identical disease occurs in cattle, called "Johne's disease" (pronounced Yo-nee's), which is caused by a bacterium, *mycobacterium avium paratuberculosis*, or "MAP." The bacterium is carried by flocks of migrating birds, which contaminate the pasturelands, causing Johne's disease in dairy cattle. MAP is then secreted in the cow's milk, finds its way into consumer milk products, and causes Crohn's disease in susceptible individuals.

Supposedly to avert a public panic, the link between Johne's disease, Crohn's disease, and milk has been suppressed by government agencies. Originally, MAP could not be seen by conventional microscopy in Crohn's disease specimens, and the theory was dismissed as fearmongering. However, with more modern DNA analysis, MAP's genetic fingerprints have been identified in practically every Crohn's disease specimen examined. Finally, the perpetrator has been uncovered.

Israel's RedHill Biopharma has developed an antibiotic cocktail - designated RHB-104 - which is effective against MAP. The results from the first Phase 3 trial, released in December 2020, were a spectacular success.

At last the real cause of Crohn's disease has been proven and an effective treatment is emerging. At last - *A Cure for Crohn's*.

BIO

A colorectal surgeon in Atlanta, GA, Dr. David Armstrong has extensive experience in treating patients with Crohn's disease. Born on a small dairy farm in North Yorkshire, England, he saw, firsthand, cattle die from Johne's disease. Emigrating to the US as a surgeon at Yale University, the Mayo Clinic, and in Atlanta GA, he saw the same wasting disease in his patients, but now it was called Crohn's disease.

Dr. Armstrong has published extensively on Crohn's disease, has developed multiple innovative surgical devices, and even developed a medication for Crohn's disease and is author of "Left Shift: How and why America is heading to second rate single payer health care". He established the first Colorectal Surgical Fellowship teaching program in the Southeastern United States. Dr. Armstrong is a Fellow of the Royal College of Surgeon, the American College of Surgeons, and the American Society of Colorectal Surgeons. He lives in Atlanta with his wife and two sons.

INDEX

Made in the USA
Monee, IL
01 July 2024

61028388R00128